The Prescription To Curing Cancer Naturally

What Doctors Won't Tell You...

Ira B. Miller

In Memory Of:

Dr. Guillermo Avecilla, who I considered the greatest family doctor and my friend. I miss him tremendously.

ISBN: 1461104513
ISBN-13: 978-1461104513

DEDICATION

This book is dedicated to my wife, Patti and to my children, Jayme and Joey. They stuck by me through thick and thin and gave me the encouragement to keep going, even when the naysayers said that I was just fooling myself if I thought that I could cure myself through these holistic methods. This is the wave of the future and I am excited to bring this method to the forefront so my kids won't have to endure what I almost had to.

ACKNOWLEDGMENTS

I would like to acknowledge Dr. Douglas Hall, my Functional Doctor, who was a great support all through this as well as a mentor and Dr. Harvey Taub, my urologist, who kept an open mind and never discouraged me to try this protocol.

CONTENTS

Introduction 7

About The Author 11

Chapter 1- **In The Beginning** 13

Chapter2- **Before The Beginning** ....…..... 21

Chapter 3- **For Your Information** ....…..... 31

Chapter 4- **More Of The Beginning** ....…..... 36

Chapter 5- **Getting Started** 52

Chapter 6- **Diet** 61

Chapter 7- **Exercise** ....…..…. 75

Chapter 8- **Herbal Treatments and Supplements** ....…... 80

Chapter 9- **More On My Experience** ....…..… 96

Chapter 10 - **Hormone Replacement Therapy** ....…. 100

Chapter 11- **Fallen People** 103

Chapter 12- **Radiation and Chemotherapy** 107

Chapter 13- **In Conclusion** ....…...111

References - ....…... 117

Index ...……..…… 119

The Truth To Curing Cancer Permanently And To A Healthy Body

INTRODUCTION

Before we begin let me first say that I am not a doctor. A doctor would probably not be writing this book as the information in this book is all about curing cancer *naturally*. There is no money to be made in the medical industry by curing yourself naturally. If everyone cured themselves naturally, the way I am about to explain to you on how I cured myself, it would greatly affect the bottom line of a lot of cancer doctors, research clinics and pharmaceutical companies; at least the ones that wouldn't change with the times. By curing cancer naturally and holistically there is a lot less need for an oncologist other than to diagnose and monitor the progress that is being made while the body heals itself. Since the pharmaceutical companies cannot patent natural herbs, diets and recipes they cannot make any money. So you won't hear about this on any T.V. commercials like you do the drugs that they make billions of dollars on. When people start realizing that you can heal yourself naturally and that information finally becomes available, like in this book, then that will take precedence rather than surgery, pharmaceuticals, radiation and/or chemotherapy. Doctors will then take a whole other approach to medicine and will then master the art of *preventative* medicine rather than *reactive* medicine. Until medical students go to school to prevent diseases rather than treat diseases books like this will not be written by doctors, only by layman such as myself who take their own time to study, literally, hundreds of hours to cure themselves. Unfortunately, until that happens, there are those that will still need the doctors that we have because there are those individuals, first of all, who don't know there is a better, more natural way. Then there are those who want a quick fix and don't want to take the time to cure themselves the natural way, the complete way; the way nature intended us to. There are also those people that are afraid to take the leap of faith that there is another way to cure themselves other than the traditional methods. Why? Because people are scared and think that the only way is the way that a medical doctor tells them. Everyone thinks that only a doctor can tell them what they need to do to cure their ailments because that doctor has been to school for years and years and interned for years in a medical environment. But, these doctors have been taught from the same books for years and there is no new methodology to treating diseases. Doctors today are stuck in a time warp and can't get out nor do they want to.

As for me, I am someone who takes a practical and common sense approach to everything that I do. I don't just take things at face value either. I don't just listen to all the experts and take that as gospel. I listen to the experts and then do my own research and after I have learned all that I can about that particular subject I then make my own determination and decisions. For example, all the doctors I talked to told me that curing my prostate cancer naturally was not possible. I have proven that it is and totally through natural holistic methods. Keep in mind, all throughout history there are those that have had this same mindset that I have and that is where all of our cutting edge inventions have come about. This is where all the new technology has come into existence and this is where even athletes have broken traditional thinking and have come up with more speed and newer tricks never before thought possible. People like me don't take "No" or "Can't" for an answer. People like me like to think "Out Of The Box"; we *live* outside of the box.

What I am about to tell you has worked for me and I am sure that if it worked for me that it can work for anyone who has cancer. That is why I have written this book. For two years I have worked on this book and for two years I have done in-depth research on the "holistic" and naturalistic approach to curing my cancer even after I was told that I could not cure my cancer this way. And I was told this not only by all my friends and family but by every one of my doctors, which there were many.

In my research I have read books and searched on the internet for everything that I could get my hands on to obtain the common sense knowledge as to <u>why</u> we get cancer as well as <u>how</u> to cure it. Knowing why we get cancer is just as important as curing it because if you just cure the cancer and don't address the reasons why we got cancer in the first place the risk of the cancer returning, and possibly with a vengeance and possibly in another area of your body, is great. Removing the cause is just as important as curing the cancer. I have known many folks that have gotten cancer and trusted the medical community to cure their cancer for them only to have the cancer removed through surgery, chemotherapy and/or radiation but only to have the cancer come back or reappear somewhere else in their bodies at a later date. So it is very important to heal your body at the cellular level not just kill the cancer and that is why I am giving you the holistic approach in this book. In case you didn't know, like I didn't know, defining the word "holistic", is this: *relating to or concerned with wholes or with complete systems rather than with the analysis of, treatment of, or dissection into parts (Merriam-Webster's Dictionary)*

So in this book I am going to give you the whole approach to curing cancer like I cured it for myself. Also, I am going to give you all the websites and book titles where I found a lot of my information. I could copy and quote everything from these websites and books and put them all in this book but then this book would be several hundred pages longer and quite boring. If you are like me you don't want to have to read through several hundred pages of facts in a book to get to the treatment of healing your cancer. If you are like me you might be saying "Just tell me how to cure my cancer and don't give me all the whys". So in this book I am going to give you just enough information from my sources on the subject at hand to help you understand why it is that I have used this source and then give you the name of the source so you can do further follow up if you like.

ABOUT THE AUTHOR

I grew up in Ft Lauderdale as a surfer/beach bum in my teen years and early twenties. Being a beach bum and partying pretty much go hand in hand. We always had parties on the beach after a great day of surfing and it was a great life. Unfortunately, it seems like that great life had caught up with me in my later years of life. It wasn't until I got into my 30's did I realize that I needed to grow up and be a productive member of society. So there were a lot of abusive years that I feel took a toll on my body and this is why I feel I contracted prostate cancer as well as skin cancer at such an early age. Actually, the skin cancer came first....I think. At least that is what I noticed first. It's not fun going to the dermatologist either and having these sores that will not go away cut and burned out of your body. The dermatologist said that the skin cancer was from too much exposure to the sun when I was younger. We did not have sun block when I was growing up. But being the out of the box thinker that I am, I came up with an ointment that healed the basil cell skin cancer lesions that were coming up in my body. No more trips to the dermatologist and no more scars on my body. So when I was told that I had prostate cancer I knew that there was a bigger problem, a possible link and there had to be another way to fight this problem.

Today, I am a building contractor and I am a very successful real estate agent in Central Florida and I use my forward thinking to further my career as well as heal myself. I want to share my story with you and the ways that you can cure your cancer once and for all like I did.

So, in this book I have done all the work. This is the Complete Guide To Curing Cancer.

The author does not directly or indirectly dispense medical advice or prescribe the use of herbs and supplements as a form of treatment for sickness without medical approval. Nutritionists and other experts in the field of health and nutrition hold widely varying views. It is not the intent of the author to diagnose or prescribe. The intent is only to offer health information to help you cooperate with your doctor in your mutual problem of building health. In the event you use this information without your doctor's approval, you are prescribing for yourself which is your constitutional right, but the publisher and author assume no responsibility.

Chapter 1

<u>**IN THE BEGINNING**</u>

When I learned that I had prostate cancer I was given four months to come back and have my prostate removed. That was the <u>only</u> option that I was given. I was only 53 years old and my doctor told me that at my age radiation was **not** the way to go. Radiation is a fast killer of cancer cells but causes a lot of damage to the surrounding nerves, tissue and muscles. He said that radiation will kill the cancer cells but it will also cause collateral damage to the nerves (over time) that serve for erections. Not only that but there is a good chance it will damage the muscles that provide urinary function too and they will suffer from the effects of radiation and cause incontinence eventually. My doctor also told me that if I did elect to go with radiation that I could not get the prostatectomy at a later date should the cancer ever come back. That was because the radiation would burn the prostate so bad that the nerves and bowel walls would be stuck to the cooked prostate and there was no way to safely remove it. If I did try to have it removed after radiation that chances of me having a colostomy bag for the rest of my life was great. I didn't like the thought of that at all. So really, my only option (at that moment) was a radical prostatectomy. I didn't even like the sound of that procedure but it sounded like I had no other choice.

I had 4 months before I had to come back for the surgery and what was I going to do with that four month grace period? My wife said that I just needed to have the prostatectomy and get it over with. She did not even remotely want me to take the chance of the cancer spreading to other areas of my body and then me dying. If you have cancer or know a loved one that does, you may be thinking this exact same way. I, on the other hand, had other thoughts. I decided to get on the internet, buy books and learn everything that I could learn about prostate cancer. There had to be another way.

When I first began my research I first learned about an experimental method of removal of the prostate called the HIFU Method that wasn't supposed to be as risky as the prostatectomy. I even called the Center For Clinical Trials because I learned that I could possibly get into a clinical trial for this HIFU method. That was the only way to get this procedure done in this country if I wanted to go this route. Other than that I had to go to another country to get it done as this was still considered an experimental procedure in this country. There was also something called the Cyber Knife but these still were all surgeries and I didn't want any part of that. Especially after I went on You Tube and saw videos of these procedures. I also saw a 60 Minutes program where a guy named John Kansius invented a radio frequency machine that killed cancer with nano-particles. This looked very promising to me but that was only experimental at the time and it was supposed to be at least another four years before the research doctor from MD Anderson, Dr Steven Curley, would be even able to start experimenting with humans. I didn't have four or more years. So I bought several books to start my journey of curing my cancer but there was one small thin book that my wife bought me called, "Natural Cancer Cures" that intrigued me the most. This and the internet led me to curing my cancer *naturally*.

Within that four month grace period I learned a lot and did a lot of experimenting. I also decided that I needed a second opinion even though I got my first biopsy at the renowned Mayo Clinic in Jacksonville, Florida; which is about two hours from where I live. I sought out the best urologist that I could find in my area. All my inquiries came down to one specific doctor, Dr. Harvey Taub. So after four months, before I went in for the prostatectomy, I went in for a second biopsy and a second opinion. I told Dr Taub about my first biopsy and showed him the results from Mayo Clinic. They were not good. Six of the ten biopsies showed signs of cancer. A couple of the cores showed seventy percent of those samples containing cancer. So I didn't have just a little bit of cancer; I had a lot. And the severity of the cancer showed Gleason Scores of mostly sevens and one six. Those weren't real good either. So I wasn't expecting much different results from what I got from Mayo but I was doing a lot of things to try and combat my cancer. Was what I was doing working? Only this second biopsy would tell.

So I went in for my second biopsy. Instead of the 10 cores that my doctor at Mayo Clinic took, Dr Taub took a twelve core sample. Now came the waiting. After a week I came back to the doctor's office for the results. As usual I waited in the lobby for what seemed like an eternity before they ever called my name. Finally I was called but it was for just the usual urine analysis, weight, blood pressure, temperature and pulse being taken. My nurse had my chart in her hand and asked me in a pleasant Latino accent, "Why do you look so worried". I had to give her a half-hearted laugh and then I said "well, it's not a good feeling having cancer and I am here now to see if anything that I have done has worked to cure my cancer and I am just worried to death about what my outcome is". She looked inside my chart and smiled and said "I don't think that you have anything to worry about" as she walked out the door. "HUH?" I looked at my wife and she looked at me and I asked, "Did you hear what she just said?". Smiling, my wife said, "I heard, she sounded like there was good news". Could it be? Could I have done what they said couldn't be done? Could I have cured my cancer? Could I have at least lessened the severity of it? Because if I didn't, and nothing has changed, then today I will be scheduling myself for surgery to have my prostate removed and I sure wasn't looking forward to that. All the complications and debilitating things that go along with that surgery scared me to death. I was too young to no longer sustain an erection and I certainly wasn't looking forward to wearing a Depends either. Now we had to sit there and wait again for the doctor and that seemed like waiting forever, too. The nurse had put my chart right outside the door in the file holder on the wall and I had all I could do not to go out there and grab that file and look at it. The waiting was killing me. I was well rehearsed by now at what I was looking at in a medical chart after all the doctor's appointments I had been to up to this point. FINALLY, the doctor came into the room. He starts off with his usual chit chat and I am thinking, "Come on Doc; give me the news". He asks how my wife is doing and he asks how I am feeling. He goes over my results to my preliminary tests that the nurse took. He then looks at me and smiles and says, "Well, I have some good news. I do not see any detectable signs of prostate cancer in this biopsy." As I was trying to process what this meant, my wife squeezed my hand so tight I thought she was going to break it. She was ecstatic at this news. I later told my brother who is a hospital administrator at the largest local hospital in town and he said that it was nothing short of a miracle of God having cured my cancer. My urologist thought that it was a miracle too but he also cautiously told me that there could be a mix-up somewhere, but he doubted it. I was thinking that there had to be a mess up somewhere too. I'm not usually a pessimist but in this case I chose not to get my hopes up until I was absolutely sure there was not a mix up somewhere. My wife, Patti, could not believe that I was not jumping up and down in hysterics and with excitement that I didn't have cancer anymore. She said that it was a lot of prayers and that with all those prayers we got to the answers that we were looking for. I was inclined to believe this, that it was divine intervention... but that Divine Intervention had *showed* us the way to a cure, not just miraculously cured me. But I couldn't help but feel that something wasn't right. To me, for the cancer to be completely gone in four months AND for my most recent Prostate Specific Antigen (PSA) tests to have *not* changed, well, I was skeptical.

So, because of my skepticism, I was not going to be convinced until I had another PSA test done because in theory, if the cancer was gone then my PSA scores should be down. Ideally, you want your PSA to be under a one and hopefully to be nonexistent. When you have a prostatectomy (removal of your prostate) your PSA scores do go down to under a 1 and are, for the most part, undetectable; for the time being that is. We'll go into that later. But, there are guys, too, who have elevated PSA scores and don't show signs of cancer. So I wasn't sure what to think at this time.

But here's the problem… I had to wait at least a month for my prostate to recover from the trauma of that last biopsy to take another PSA test to get non-skewed PSA score results. Because of the trauma of the biopsy, my PSA would most likely be way up. Your PSA goes up just by having sex the night before a PSA test is done, so I can imagine what it would be like after a biopsy. As of right now it has only been a week. So now I had to wait another three long weeks for it to be a month before I could go get my blood drawn again for a good PSA test. I waited exactly a month and then I got the PSA test and then another week later to get the results. The waiting in all this is very tolling. But then came the results and the test told the story. My PSA was the same as it has always been. It was a 1.9. "Oh no!" I was pretty upset at this point. What was I to think? In my mind there were only two scenarios. Either Mayo Clinic, where I had gotten my first biopsy and the news I had prostate cancer, had gotten my first biopsy results mixed up with someone else's and I never did have cancer or my local pathologist got the second biopsy mixed up with someone else's and I did still have a severe case of prostate cancer on my hands. In either scenario there was no book to be written. I had not cured (my) prostate cancer. I either never had it to start with or I still had it to the extremes that my first biopsy said I had it, all according to my PSA test results.

Dr Taub and I had already decided that we were going to do a third biopsy in a month and the third biopsy was only a week away...and then the truth. It was either that or have a DNA test done on both samples to make sure that both samples were mine. Unfortunately, DNA tests were out of the question because it would cost about $5000 for the DNA test and no one was willing to pay for the test and I didn't have the money to either. So, since my insurance company was willing to pay the many thousands of dollars for me to have another biopsy (which was more than if they would have paid for the DNA testing, which didn't make sense, but then again, insurance companies never do make sense) my only other option was another biopsy. But, for added measures, Dr. Taub sent for my specimen samples from Mayo. Mayo had them stored away. Dr. Taub sent those Mayo samples and the samples that he got back from his lab to a different independent lab and the results came back just the same. The Mayo samples showed high signs of prostatic cancer and Dr. Taub's sample showed no signs of prostate cancer.

So the day came for my third biopsy. I was finally going to find out if Mayo messed up or if Dr. Taub messed up. For my third biopsy, instead of his normal 12 core sample biopsy, Dr Taub suggested that he should do 24 core samples. I didn't like the thought of that. If you have ever had a biopsy done you will know what I am talking about. The 12 core samples that he took last time were bad enough but we had to know once and for all so I said go ahead, it sounded like the best idea. Besides, something humorous came to mind. It seemed at this rate, if I did still have cancer, I was going to get rid of it just by having all these biopsies (which could never really happen by the way). Anyway, he went ahead and did the 24 core samples and sent them off. Then came the long wait; again with the waiting…

After a week I got the test results AND a third scenario. A Third Scenario? Yes, a third scenario. The cancer was still there… there just wasn't that much of it left. It seems that the second biopsy didn't find the little remaining cancer that the third biopsy had found and therefore it was thought that there was no cancer left. The PSA test (and my Mayo doctor by the way) told me that there *was* still cancer there. Dr Taub said it just wasn't as severe as the first test that Mayo had done showed. So, what I was doing was working after all. Mayo didn't screw up, my pathologist here locally didn't screw up and my cancer appeared to be *almost* gone. Only two of the 24 cores showed signs of cancer and very little of it according to the percentage of cancer that was in the each core. I thought "Hurray, let's keep up the good work and get rid of the rest of this cancer" and get to writing this book.

So, in this book you will read how I defeated and cured my prostate cancer and not with radiation and not by surgically removing my prostate which is about the only other clinically proven methods that will be told to you.

I read a book recently where the author claimed to have cured his prostate cancer 100% holistically but when you read that book you find out that he had chemotherapy and radiation first. I have had none of that. I cured my cancer 100%, holistically, naturally and with common over the counter herbs, supplements and a little heard of, special, sulphurated protein recipe. Not only will you read how I got rid of my prostate cancer, there is a lot of other valuable and knowledgeable information on diet, losing weight, anti-aging, and cures for other problems that I had like acid reflux disease and skin cancer. Please read on and enjoy a healthy life.

Chapter 2

BEFORE THE BEGINNING

For two years, before I learned that I had prostate cancer, I was seeing a Functional Doctor named Dr. Douglas Hall. For those of you that don't know what a "Functional" Doctor is they are also known as Anti-Aging Doctors. I had gone to my Internal Medicine family physician years before and told him that I was feeling run down. No matter how much sleep I was getting I was still tired and faded fast toward the end of the work day. I tried exercising, which was a chore since I was so tired at the end of the day and that didn't seem to help. I was gaining weight and my stomach was really starting to gain size and protrude. My size 33 pants were getting really tight. I saw some pictures of me on the beach and I was repulsed at what I saw. What was happening to me? I was getting old and fat. I hated the thought. I had been thin my whole life and I was not used to this. I needed to do something about that. I was always interested in longevity anyway and I had read and watched TV programs even as far back as when I was an adolescent and a teenager. I could remember the pioneers of functional medicine, Dirk Pearson and Sandy Shaw, talking about anti-aging way back when. And then upon further investigation I even read that my problem may possibly be that my Adrenal Glands were burnt out. "Oh Man, I am a mess". I needed help and I needed it quick.

Then I saw a program on 60 Minutes. It was about an Anti-Aging movement. "Oh My Gosh, this is what I had been looking for!" It featured Dr. Alan Mintz and his company called Cenegenics Medical Institute. I called Dr. Mintz and he personally called me back and invited me to come to Las Vegas to meet him. I was very excited about going out there to meet Dr. Mintz. However, I did learn that there was a Cenegenics Medical Institute in Charleston, South Carolina that was driving distance for me. So I decided to drive the 5 hours from Florida to Charleston to meet with one of his colleagues at one of their national branch offices instead. His colleague's name was Dr. Mickey Barber. She filled me in on what Cenegenics was all about. This was great but, for me at the time, I thought that it was too expensive. They were talking about $3500 initial work ups and then over $500 a month to be on this program properly. But again, I was desperate and I was getting ready to at least try it. I was thinking that if this works then I will more than make up for the expense with the extra work I could accomplish with all the energy that this would give me. Plus, just plain feeling better; how do you put a price on that? It is all about quality of life.

When I came home I told my neighbor, Jason, who happened to be a pharmaceutical rep, where I just came from and what I was getting ready to do. He then told me that a good friend of ours father, who just happened to be a *gynecologist*, was in the field of Functional Medicine now and seeing male patients. I don't know. I think that I would feel p-r-e-t-t-y silly sitting in a waiting room with 10 women waiting for their pelvic exam. I made the appointment anyway as *desperate times require desperate measures*. This was too important to me.

When I got to the office I asked myself how bad could it be. Maybe the women in there will think that I am just waiting on my wife. I'm sure there have been other guys that have done that before, right? They have gone to the gynecologist with their wife and waited out in the waiting room? On hindsight…. maybe not. But, I gathered my courage and I walked into the office and sat down. There I was, sitting in the waiting room. I looked at a lady on my right and sure enough, just like I figured would happen, she was staring at me. I just smiled, looked her in the eyes and nodded my head. She looked back down at her magazine. I then looked away and there was another lady staring at me. I could just see what she was thinking, "What in the world is HE doing here… and by himself?" "Oh Brother!" I was then called and I got up and just smiled at both of them and nodded as I walked to the office door. Holy Cow, I am so glad that I didn't have to wait out there too long. I think that Dr Hall must have been sensitive to the idea of male patients waiting in a gynecologist's office.

I went in and met Dr Hall for the very first time. Dr Hall was in his early 60's although you couldn't tell it. He was a good looking guy for his age, no wrinkles to speak of on his face and you could tell that he worked out and was in good shape. I told him my problems and he smiled a huge toothy grin and with all the confidence in the world said, "Don't worry, this isn't a problem. We'll have you taken care of in no time. I have just the answer." He prescribed a saliva test and blood work from Spectra Cell Laboratories. I laughed inside; was I was finally on my way to Peter Pan land? Then, what seemed like forever took 2 weeks to get my results back. I couldn't wait. I was ready for Step 2. Dr. Hall's office called me and told me that my results were back and we set an appointment for the following week. I had to wait a whole 'nother week to get this in gear? Oh nooo…. But anyway, the day finally came for me to meet up with my hero, my savior, again. As it turned out he was my savior in more ways than one.

Months before, at my annual Executive Physical at Mayo Clinic in Jacksonville, I was telling my doctor there about the horrible acid reflux I was having for the past couple of years. Whenever I went out to dinner and overate or had a couple of margaritas I had severe pain in my solar plexus. This was crazy. They first did an endoscopy along with my colonoscopy to make sure that I didn't have any esophageal erosion or Barrett's esophagus (Pre-cancer of the esophagus). Luckily I did not. That was my first scare with potential cancer. There were 2 surgical solutions that my brother Marc told me about, who was CEO for a medical billing company at the time in Asheville, North Carolina. Today, he is Senior Vice President of Physicians Services at a local hospital here in Ocala, Florida. They were procedures called Laparoscopic Fundoplication or a Nissen Fundoplication. This is where they cut you open and tie your trachea and esophagus together or something like that. "Oh, forget that!" No surgery for this guy. Instead I elected to go with the typical prescribed solution of Prilosec and Nexium. That was fine as long as my insurance was paying for it because of how expensive it was but then Prilosec went over the counter and then I ended up pulling all that money out of my pocket anyway.

Back to Dr Hall's Spectra Cell Laboratories' blood test, he started out talking a million miles an hour and he talked about technical and medical things that I never in a million years could understand what he was talking about. He was telling me about what cells are made up of and how they worked and what the chemical reaction is when you introduce this supplement and that supplement into your system. He had all these flip charts in a notebook and these charts looked like a company flow chart. This tied to that and that caused this to do something else and down the chart he went..... Oh man, it made my head spin. I thought to myself, "surely he doesn't think that I know what the heck he is talking about? I'm just going to have to do my best to stay up with him the best that I can". He lost me and every other meeting that I had ever had with him after that the same thing would happen. I would go to see him to this day saying to myself, "I am going to listen to him intently and he is not going to lose me", but he does every time. Fortunately, each time I see him now I have learned a little more and each time it takes him longer and longer to lose me but eventually he still does. I will get there one day though, where he won't lose me.... One Day.....

Then he got to my results. He said that everything looked fine with the blood test except I was low in Pantothenic Acid. Huh? I never heard of that; much less was able to pronounce Pant-o-then-ic. I eventually was able to get that word to just roll off my tongue as I learned that the lack of it was the cause of my acid reflux. Can you believe that? A big huge research clinic such as Mayo didn't find that I was deficient in Pantothenic Acid and that was the cure to my acid reflux disease. Halleluiah! What a hero Dr Hall was. But it gets even better.

We then went into what the saliva test had to say. My testosterone levels were in the toilet. <u>Severely</u> depressed levels and I needed to get on supplemental testosterone right away. Yay… I couldn't wait. I started out with the testosterone 'cream' that you squeeze out of a syringe onto your inner forearm and then rub onto your inner thigh. It comes in a 10cc syringe and I was using 1cc a day for 5 days so each syringe contained a 2 week supply. It had to be compounded at a local pharmaceutical lab and I would receive a 6 week supply. No shots too! What a plus. I was not looking forward to having to get injections every week which is what I thought I was going to have to go through. This was getting better all the time. Unbelievable! I was rubbing this cream on the inside of my leg once a day in the morning for 5 days and then quit on the weekends. You would not believe how much better that made me feel. It was just what the doctor ordered (Pun Intended). I was a new man.

It wasn't like a light switch was turned on. I didn't have an instant rush or instant high energy but I felt normal again. I had my normal energy back. I was thinking so much clearer and could actually remember things again. Before I got on the testosterone replacement I was missing appointments and meetings all the time and I could never even remember my customers' names, who I had sold homes to. How embarrassing is that? But now I could remember people's names as I met them walking down the street, which seemed miraculous at the time. How great that felt!

I stayed on the testosterone cream for about 8 months. I got into working out with weights. I was jogging 3 miles

3 times a week. I was getting into shape, feeling better and really enjoying life again. I then read Suzanne Somers' book called "Ageless". It talked about testosterone replacement as well as human growth hormones. Growth Hormones?... Hmmmm... This sounded interesting. Was I ready to move on to the next step; the next level? I asked Dr Hall about getting on HGH and he told me that he didn't use HGH as that was banned for use by the federal government but there was a product out there called Sermorelin and it was a GHRH. That stands for Growth Hormone Releasing Hormone. This drug actually caused your pituitary gland to release higher levels of growth hormone naturally. There was no risk for overdosing on Growth Hormones with Sermorelin and the theory was that your body would be producing growth hormones like it was when you were in your twenties to thirties. Oh man, what I wouldn't give to feel like I felt when I was in my twenties and thirties. I was already feeling good on the testosterone but could it get even better, I wondered? Sermorelin was not cheap. It was $500 for 2 bottles that lasted for a month. AND.... It was injectable only. Ut oh... That is not where I really wanted to go. No needles for this guy... But, if I wanted to go all the way and do all that was available to me to stay feeling young I HAD to do it. So, thus started my delve into the world of injections.

Well actually, years ago when I was around 34 years old I worked in a gym and got with guys that were *shooting* steroids and I got into that as well. I was doing just 1cc of testosterone in the butt once a week but boy did my workouts get awesome. I went from bench pressing 185 pounds max to 275 in about 3 months. I was seeing that 315 pinnacle (3-45 pound plates on each side of the bar).

That was my goal. I never made it though. The guys quit the gym that I was working at and I couldn't get the "test" anymore. Down I went in weight. Oh man, talk about depression setting in. I was lucky to be lifting 225 lbs. (2 plates on each side of the bar). It was better than where I started out but….. That was my first experience with testosterone and injections. In hindsight, I have a feeling that that experience with injecting testosterone may have caused my testicles to shut down and caused my situation with the low testosterone that I am experiencing today. I would not recommend that anyone take steroids. The risk far outweighs the advantages. Then there is the "crash" you get when you get off of them too. It's just not worth it in my opinion.

Dr. Hall gave me some needles and told me where to order the Sermorelin. Wow, he gave me some daggers. He gave me a handful of 25 gauge 1½ inch syringes. OH… My... G--… "I have to stick myself with these needles and WHERE; in the fatty tissue of my thigh or my stomach (called subcutaneous)?" THAT took some doing. When I got the Sermorelin I got out my needles and mixed the two products together as you have to mix 3 ml's of sterile water with the powdered solution. I drew up .2 ml's into the syringe and I was ready. I sat there for 15 minutes trying to do this. There wasn't much fatty tissue there but the leg seemed better than the stomach. I pinched as much fatty tissue as I could get. I started to do it, then… no no no no… I couldn't do it….I tried it again and no no no no, I couldn't do it. Finally, I plunged the needle down and wham…. I did it. I couldn't believe it. I was doing it but it burned. I didn't really like this but for $500 per month of Sermorelin and getting back to my youthful exaltation, I was going to do it come hell or high water. I *was* doing it. Come to find out, though, I didn't have to use these daggers that Dr. Hall had given me. I found out that I could use 30 gauge needles that were 5/8" long that were actually insulin needles since Sermorelin is water based.... muuuch better.

I stayed on the Sermorelin for close to a year. I had difficulty getting it sometimes. Only certain pharmacies would carry it. One time, the one pharmacy I always got it from said that they were no longer carrying Sermorelin. OH NO! You're kidding... I panicked. I had to have my Fountain of Youth. I called Dr. Halls office and told him that our pharmacy no longer carried Sermorelin. What was he (me) going to do? He suggested another pharmacy and I was back in business. But it didn't seem like it was the same formula and I started to think that I was becoming obsessed with this when I panicked because the last pharmacy didn't offer this anymore. Also, I was thinking that this really isn't making me feel any better than when I first felt when I got on the testosterone. So I decided to go off the Sermorelin and in reality.... I don't think that I felt any different when I did go off of it.

Now that I was used to giving myself injections I asked Dr Hall about giving myself injections of testosterone instead of the cream every day. He said that this is what he does because he gives this to himself once a week and then doesn't have to worry about it anymore for the week. The only thing is you can only stay on the injectable testosterone for up to 5 weeks and then have to go off of it and get on something called HCG or Human Chorionic Gonadotropin. This drug prompts the testicles to start producing testosterone on their own because excessive use of testosterone will cause the testicles to shut down production. So as to prevent the testicles from atrophying this cycling must take place. I was a bit worried that this HCG might cause cancer. So I don't know if I liked the idea of *injecting* testosterone. The HCG was an injectable prescription as well. This was easier, of course, because it was water based and I was able to use much smaller needles to inject the solution into my body like I discovered I could use with Sermorelin; much more comfortable to use. The testosterone is oil based and the liquid will not pass through those 30 gauge needles so you have to use a thicker 25 gauge needle. I ultimately did get on the injectable testosterone and the HCG program. It seemed to me like there were some peaks and valleys doing it this way though so I eventually went back to the cream. I never did the patch and I think once I get back on the testosterone program that I may look into that.

Once again, I want to note that a lot of this information comes from the book "Ageless" by Suzanne Somers. It might sound crazy that I would acknowledge someone who played Chrissy on 3's Company back in the '70's but she makes a good point and talks a lot of sense in that book. Not only that, but her findings are based on a lot of interviews with cutting edge doctors. These are the doctors of the anti-aging movement. But that is for later on in this book. I would recommend reading this book.

Chapter 3

FOR YOUR INFORMATION

Since 2001, every year I would go to Mayo Clinic in Jacksonville for an Executive Physical. An Executive Physical is where you would spend a day (or two if you were having a colonoscopy) at Mayo Clinic having a battery of tests done. At the end of your tests you would see your assigned personal physician and he would go over your results with you. It is a wonderful way to get completely checked out and then have all the results that same day. I would highly recommend that everyone start getting a physical at a major medical institution, if possible, and track your results. To younger people, it also gives you a baseline to go off of in subsequent years as you grow older. This way your doctor can look back at your baselines from years past and help you supplement your hormones to get you back to that youthful state. Spread the word. Get your Baselines... Very Important...

I told my doctor there, Doctor Rodriguez, what I was doing. He was not a big fan of me doing testosterone hormone replacement therapy. He tried to discourage both me and my wife; telling my wife to talk me out of it. He said that it will cause me to get prostate cancer, or fuel it if nothing else, if I ever did contract prostate cancer. I said "Doctor Rodriguez, I would rather have quality of life rather than quantity of life. So I'm asking you to just make sure that I stay healthy and to keep an eye out to make sure that prostate cancer or any cancer for that matter does not sneak up on me". About 2007 he said that my PSA levels looked like they were getting elevated and while they were still in the safe range he still had cause for concern. I assured him that the only reason that my PSA levels were going up was most likely because of the testosterone I was taking and I didn't think that I had anything to worry about.

The next year, in 2008, my PSA levels had gone up even more. This gave him even more cause for concern and he highly suggested that I get a biopsy just to make sure that I didn't have prostate cancer. Hmmm. So I asked him, "Just exactly what does a prostate biopsy entail?" He told me that it is where they stick a probe up your rectum and insert a spring loaded gun that has a long needle on the end that propels this needle through your colon and into your prostate 10 to 12 times to take out tissue samples of your prostate. Well... I don't think so.... Not when my PSA levels are in the safe range of a 2.0 PSA. THAT'S just not going to happen. I still think that my levels had gone up due to the testosterone hormone replacement that I was on; even more so now. I guess that I was in denial.... You know.... "Denial ... That River That Runs Through Egypt"? Bad Joke!

Well, Dr. Rodriguez tells me that he is going to have an endocrinologist talk to me. This is a hormone specialist. No problem. I go down to where this endocrinologists' office is and we meet and we talk. The beautiful thing about going to Mayo is that everything is right there on site and at the disposal of the attending physician. That's how I got in to see this specialist so quickly. The endocrinologist was not a big fan of hormone replacement therapy either. He told me that what I was doing was dangerous and he did not recommend it. I told him that I had a much better quality of life while I was on this and that it just seemed logical to me that if guys in their 20's and 30's had higher levels of testosterone why not me? If guys in their 20's and 30's healed quicker, had bigger muscles, had a higher energy level, and looked better AND didn't have prostate cancer then I didn't see any reason why I couldn't go back to that period of time when I was like that too. He didn't really have an answer for that. I guess maybe it made sense to him logically; it just flew in the face of what he was taught in medical school.

Dr Rodriguez then scheduled me to talk to the urologist about a biopsy. At this point my PSA was wavering between a 2 and a 2.5. But again, the big concern was that it had gone up in 2 years from a .8 to these levels. PSA levels are supposed to stay under a one or if nothing else, not go up every year. So I went to the urologist and he looked at my records. He highly recommended that I get the biopsy as well. I made him a deal. I said that if my PSA levels come down to under a 2 then I am not going to have the biopsy. He said deal. So we made the appointment and scheduled the biopsy and scheduled the PSA test for the same day. Like I said, the beautiful thing about Mayo is that everything is right there. You don't have to wait days or weeks for your results. You know within hours. I was convinced that the testosterone was the culprit so I got off all the testosterone and all my supplements just to make sure that nothing was causing a false reading on the PSA test. I did this for a month and then came back to Mayo. We did the PSA test and then two hours later I was up in the urologist's room getting prepped for the biopsy. I said "Whoa, wait a minute. I have a deal with Dr Theil that if my PSA levels were under a 2 that we would not do the biopsy today. The prep nurse checked with Dr. Theil and Dr. Theil confirmed that. My PSA levels were at 1.9. So I said that I am going to hold off and we can continue to monitor things.

I still felt that there was no way that someone like me who exercised, ate a hand full of vitamins and supplements twice a day, who just turned 53 years old, could possibly have prostate cancer. Although, my dad did die of rectal cancer; but he was 72. I then had Dr Hall do another blood test on me to test my testosterone levels and my PSA while he was at it about a month later. The results came back that my testosterone levels were too high because I had gone to see another Functional Doctor just to get a second opinion on my testosterone levels and that doctor had upped my testosterone intake as well as put me on a different kind of testosterone. I had forgotten that there were different kinds of testosterone. He told me that the kind that Dr. Hall had me on was the cheap stuff and that I needed to up my cc intake and get on testosterone cyponate. So I did. But Patti, my wife, didn't like this guy for some reason. She said that she didn't have a good feeling about him and I have learned in my 12 years of marriage (at that time) that if she didn't have a good feeling about something then she was usually right. So, I went back to Dr. Hall and sure enough my testosterone levels were too high. He also introduced me to "Free" PSA readings. This was the first time that I had heard about Free PSA. It apparently was a better indicator of prostate cancer than just the PSA levels. While my PSA levels were relatively in the safe range my Free PSA levels were not. Those readings are supposed to be high; the opposite of the regular PSA readings. Mine were very low and Dr. Hall said that by these readings I had a 28% chance of having prostate cancer. My readings were at 13. I asked him what his were. He said that his were around 58. I asked what he would do if he were me. He said that he would have a biopsy as soon as possible to make sure that I was not "pouring gasoline on the fire". This alarmed me when he said that. I had listened to Dr. Hall up to now so there was no reason to stop at this point. So I immediately called Mayo and scheduled the biopsy.

Chapter 4

<u>MORE OF THE BEGINNING</u>

Mayo got me in in about 3 weeks. I went in and had 10 core samples taken. This was on a Wednesday. They were going to try and have my results back by Friday so I didn't have to suffer waiting all weekend to hear the results. I didn't get the call until Monday morning though. Dr. Theil called me and told me the terrifying news. Trust me, you never forget where you were on the day and time that you hear devastating news like that. Do you remember where you were at the time of 9/11? If you are reading this book, chances are that you have cancer and you know what I am talking about.

When I found out that I had cancer I was horrified….. I was stunned… My whole world was rocked. I HAD CANCER???? I couldn't believe it. I lived a fast life in my early adulthood. I did party a lot but I thought that I had made up for all that with my lifestyle that I had chosen as of late. I started working out with weights in my mid-thirties. I had turned to herbal supplements when I joined the anti-aging movement. I really turned things around. I felt so much better and I became a productive member of society. I worked hard and wanted to make something out of my life. Little did I know that if you don't do any intervention that what you did over your lifetime *will* eventually catch up with you.

What do I mean by intervention? Basically, I mean by cleansing out all those impurities that your body accumulated over your lifetime. Also, you may have heard how the medical community will tell you about skin damage from prolonged exposure to the sun. It never made any sense to me that what I did in my younger years would stay in my system and linger until I got of an older age and then come out with a vengeance. But supposedly, by today's thinking, skin cancer is caused by the sun exposure that you received when you were younger. This may be true. I have a tendency to believe that skin cancer is more inherent rather than caused by what I did 30 - 40 years ago as a youth. But for the sake of argument I am not a doctor so I went with this theory…. Just in case.

So I thought, "Well, if this was the case, that what I did in my earlier years will catch up with me in my later years, what can I do about it now"? I was asking myself "had my partying days caught up with me and that has caused my prostate cancer? Had pollution in the water and air accumulated in my body and caused this? Were the pesticides that were used on my lawn or in my home to kill bugs the culprit?" I need to see what I can do about this. There has to be a way where I can reverse or annul this. This is where I decided that I was going to start curing my cancer myself.

The first thing that I had settled on in my mind was that the cancer must have been triggered by something in my system since getting prostate cancer at 53 is not too common. I also thought that I was not going to do any good in trying to cure my cancer if what caused it or triggered it was still aggravating the situation. So the very first thing that I thought that I needed to do was to purge myself of any and all impurities that I could. This was done by colon cleansing, cellular cleansing, as well cleansing of heavy metals. A colon cleanser for two reasons: One to remove any impurities, toxins and poisons that may be lodged and clogging up my intestines over the years and possibly causing a contamination of my body and the other was for providing a clean intestine to allow for better absorption of the supplements that I was getting ready to take. "Cellular" cleansing was done using Essiac Tea. Bentonite was used to take out any heavy metals that may be in my body. Most heavy metals are toxic to our system and need to be removed. It was my opinion that if cancer was in my body it had to have started either with the toxins and impurities that are in my colon or the heavy metals or both.

With the cause gone now I could then take on the task of curing the cancer. How was I going to find out about doing that? Everyone told me that I needed to just go ahead and have "The Surgery"; the Radical Prostatectomy. Well, if there was any way that I was going to avoid THAT I was going to do it. There was no way that I wanted that surgery. I had heard some horror stories about that; namely incontinence and impotence. That was not for me. I was not going to risk walking around in an adult Depends the rest of my life and neither did I want to take the chance of never having an erection again. I was way too young to stop having sex now. I had just discovered Viagra and it was great. Cialis turned out to be even better. I wanted to keep going and enjoy life just the way that I have been enjoying it up until now. Also, I discovered that having the prostatectomy is not always a 100% cure for prostate cancer. In many instances, there have been men that have had the prostatectomy and years later discovered that their PSA was going up again due to prostatic cancer cells having escaped the capsule of the prostate and lodged somewhere else in the body. There have been many men, they say about 50% within 5 years, where prostate cancer returns even after having the prostatectomy and it usually ends up in the bones. This was an important fact and needed to be given much consideration.

So what was I to do…? Well, first and foremost I consider myself a practical thinker and I have a great deal of common sense. So what is the most practical and common sense way to approach finding a cure for this prostate cancer? Reading and research! I wanted to find a way to make sure that I cured my prostate cancer naturally and have a comfort level that it will be gone for good. So if I can cure it naturally then I don't have to worry that any escaped. Also, somewhere down the road I won't have to worry that I had the surgery for nothing as it is growing in my bones or liver or somewhere else. Curing it holistically means that I killed it and it is gone for good. So let's start at the beginning to learn how I cured my cancer and healed my body so it never returns.

Urology Procedure   MILLER, IRA - 5-532-████

Result Type: Urology Procedure
Result Date: January 21, 2009 12:00 AM
Result Status: Auth (Verified)
Performed By: Thiel MD, David D on January 21, 2009 3:09 PM
Verified By: Thiel MD, David D on January 23, 2009 8:50 AM
Encounter Info: 3091923, MAYO, MCJ Patient, 7/25/2001 -

MILLER, IRA MR.
5-532-████████

01/21/2009   David D. Thiel, M.D.
         1356

PREOPERATIVE DIAGNOSIS
Elevated prostate-specific antigen (PSA).

POSTOPERATIVE DIAGNOSIS
Elevated prostate-specific antigen (PSA).

PROCEDURE
Transrectal ultrasound-guided prostate biopsy.

DESCRIPTION OF PROCEDURE
After proper consent was obtained and patient identified as Ira Miller, he
was brought into the biopsy suite and placed in the left lateral decubitus
position at which time his prostate was topically anesthetized in the
standard fashion. The transrectal ultrasound probe was introduced in his
rectum. The prostate was anesthetized with 1% lidocaine for a total of 8 mL
on the right and left hand sides of the prostate at the junction of the
seminal vesicles and the base of the prostate. Biopsies were taken x10 in
the standard fashion, including the right and left, base, mid, apices and
lateral horns. The patient tolerated the procedure well. Gentamicin 80 mg
I.M. x1 was given. He was given Levaquin 250 mg p.o. daily for 3 days.

FINDINGS
The prostatic size was 28.6 grams. There were no abnormal hyperechoic or
hypoechoic lesions in the prostate.

DDT:mm
D:01/21/2009 15:09
T:01/22/2009 11:24
REVISED DATE: TRANS:1823

Printed by: Coles, Connie L   Page 1 of 2
Printed on: 2/9/2009 3:30 PM   (Continued)

Urology Procedure   MILLER, IRA - 5-532████

Completed Action List:
* Perform by Thiel MD, David D on January 21, 2009 3:09 PM
* Transcribe by Mebee, Michele on January 22, 2009 11:24 AM
* Sign by Thiel MD, David D on January 23, 2009 8:50 AM January 23, 2009 8:50 AM
* Verify by Thiel MD, David D on January 23, 2009 8:50 AM

41

Surgical Path Final   MILLER, IRA - 5-532-███

* Final Report *

Result Type:	Surgical Path Final
Result Date:	January 21, 2009 3:52 PM
Result Status:	Auth (Verified)
Result Title:	SurgPath Final
Verified By:	Nakhleh MD, Raouf E on January 22, 2009 1:22 PM
Encounter Info:	3091923, MAYO, MCJ Patient, 7/25/2001 -

* Final Report *

GROSS DESCRIPTION

A) In formalin labeled "left apex" is a 1.2 cm cylindrical fragment of gray/tan soft tissue. All blocked labeled as A1.

B) In formalin labeled "left mid" is a 1.0 cm cylindrical fragment of gray/tan soft tissue. All blocked labeled as B1.

C) In formalin labeled "left base" is a 1.0 cm cylindrical fragment of gray/tan soft tissue. All blocked labeled as C1.

D) In formalin labeled "right apex" is a 0.8 cm cylindrical fragment of gray/tan soft tissue. All blocked labeled as D1.

E) In formalin labeled "right mid" is a 1.0 cm cylindrical fragment of gray/tan soft tissue. All blocked labeled as E1.

F) In formalin labeled "right base" are two cylindrical fragments of gray/tan soft tissue ranging in size from 0.3 cm up to 0.5 cm in greatest dimension. All blocked labeled as F1.

G) In formalin labeled "left proximal" is a 1.0 cm cylindrical fragment of gray/tan soft tissue. All blocked labeled as G1.

H) In formalin labeled "right proximal" is a 0.9 cm cylindrical fragment of gray/tan soft tissue. All blocked labeled as H1.

I) In formalin labeled "left distal" is a 1.0 cm cylindrical fragment of gray/tan soft tissue. All blocked labeled as I1.

J) In formalin labeled "right distal" are two cylindrical fragments of gray/tan soft tissue ranging in size up to 0.8 cm in greatest dimension. All blocked labeled as J1.
MEC/blb

SPECIMEN RECEIVED

42

Surgical Path Final

MILLER, IRA - 5-532-████

TRNB LOBE PROSTATE
  A) LEFT APEX   F) RIGHT BASE
  B) LEFT MID   G) LEFT PROXIMAL
  C) LEFT BASE   H) RIGHT PROXIMAL
  D) RIGHT APEX   I) LEFT DISTAL
  E) RIGHT MID   J) RIGHT DISTAL

FINAL DIAGNOSIS
  A) Prostate, left apex, needle biopsy: Negative for malignancy.

  B) Prostate, left mid, needle biopsy: Negative for malignancy.

  C) Prostate, left base, needle biopsy: Adenocarcinoma, Gleason score 3+4=7,
     involving 20% of tissue.

  D) Prostate, right apex, needle biopsy: Adenocarcinoma, Gleason score 3+3=6,
     involving 30% of tissue.

  E) Prostate, right mid, needle biopsy: Adenocarcinoma, Gleason score 3+4=7,
     involving 65% of tissue.

  F) Prostate, right base, needle biopsy: Adenocarcinoma, Gleason score 3+4=7,
     involving 70% of tissue.

  G) Prostate, left proximal, needle biopsy: Benign prostatic tissue.

  H) Prostate, right proximal, needle biopsy: Adenocarcinoma, Gleason score 3+4=7,
     involving <5% of tissue.

  I) Prostate, left distal, needle biopsy: Adenocarcinoma, Gleason score 3+4=7,
     involving approximately 10% of tissue.

  J) Prostate, right distal, needle biopsy: Benign prostatic tissue.
  REN/hw

Signature Line
    REN:HLW   Raouf E Nakhleh, MD
    01/22/2009   ~electronic signature~

Printed by: Coles, Connie L
Printed on: 2/9/2009 3:30 PM

Page 2 of 3
(Continued)

43

Surgical Path Final   MILLER, IRA - 5-532-█████

Completed Action List:
* Verify by Nakhleh MD, Raouf E on January 22, 2009 1:22 PM
* Order by Thiel MD, David D on January 21, 2009 3:52 PM
* Review by Thiel MD, David D on January 26, 2009 9:39 AM

44

Bone Scan

MILLER, IRA - 5-532-█████

* Final Report *

Result Type:	Bone Scan
Result Date:	January 29, 2009 1:39 PM
Result Status:	Auth (Verified)
Performed By:	Dalton MD, Jon N on January 29, 2009 1:39 PM
Verified By:	Dalton MD, Jon N on January 29, 2009 2:31 PM
Encounter info:	3091923, MAYO, MCJ Patient, 7/25/2001 -

* Final Report *

Name : Ira Miller
MRN : 05-532-085-7

Ordering Physician : 1356
Creation Date : 01/29/2009
Performed At : Radiology 2nd Floor MCJ
Indications : 185 Ca Prostate - Cancer,, ,NA,
29 Jan 2009 2:31PM *** Final ***
NM Bone Scan WB
Radionuclide Bone Scan:
History: Prostate cancer
22.0 mCi Tc-99m MDP was injected intravenously per protocol followed by
planar imaging of the entire skeleton in anterior and posterior
projections.
No comparisons.
Findings: No foci of increased activity suspicious for osseous
metastatic disease. Increased uptake in the hips, knees, ankles, and
left great toe consistent with degenerative changes. Physiologic uptake
is seen in the kidneys and bladder.
This report was dictated by Dr. A. Smith after review with Dr. Dalton.
A.R. Smith, M.D.
J.N. Dalton, MD

Completed Action List:
* Order by Thiel MD, David D on January 29, 2009 1:39 PM
* Verify by Dalton MD, Jon N on January 29, 2009 2:31 PM
* Perform by Dalton MD, Jon N on January 29, 2009 1:39 PM
* Endorse by Thiel MD, David D on January 30, 2009 2:53 PM

Printed by:	Coles, Connie L	Page 1 of 1
Printed on:	2/9/2009 3:30 PM	(End of Report)

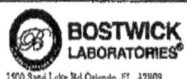

BOSTWICK LABORATORIES®

2500 Sand Lake Rd Orlando, FL 32809
Phone 407-888-1051   Fax 407-856-0533   www.bostwicklaboratories.com

BL09-0102-0003421

|||||||||||||||||||||||||||||||||

Date Collected: 04/23/2009
Date Received: 04/23/2009
Date Reported: 04/27/2009

Name:	Ira B Miller
SSN:	▬▬▬
Date of Birth:	▬▬▬
Requisition #:	BU90004239
Phone:	▬▬▬

Sex: Male
Age: 53

Harvey C Taub, M.D.
Associates for Urology Care
1901 SE 18th Ave Building 300
Ocala, FL 34471

Phone: (352) 351-1313
Fax: (352) 351-1927

Provided ICD-9 codes: 185, EUS

The specimen is received in 12 vials containing pink-tan, 0.1 cm diameter prostate biopsies in formalin; submitted in toto.

Site	Length
(A) Right Apex racemase,34B-E12,p63 AND c-myc	1.7 cm
(B) Right Mid	1.3 cm (Stringy)
(C) Right Base	1.2 cm (Stringy)
(D) Right Lat Apex	1.4 cm (Stringy, Fragmented)
(E) Right Lat Mid	1.1 cm (Stringy, Fragmented)
(F) Right Lat Base	1.0 cm (Stringy, Fragmented)
(G) Left Apex racemase,34B-E12,p63 AND c-myc	1.6 cm
(H) Left Mid	1.5 cm (Stringy)
(I) Left Base racemase,34B-E12,p63 AND c-myc	1.1 cm (Fragmented)
(J) Left Lat Apex	1.4 cm (Fragmented)
(K) Left Lat Mid	1.2 cm (Fragmented)
(L) Left Lat Base	1.1 cm (Fragmented)

Specimens received on blue sponges.

HGPIN ▨▨▨   SUSPICIOUS ▨▨▨   MALIGNANT ▬▬

PROSTATE, NEEDLE BIOPSIES

(A)	Right Apex:	Benign prostatic tissue. Immunostains for basal cell-specific high molecular weight keratin (34BE12), p63, racemase and c-myc support this diagnosis.
(B)	Right Mid:	Benign prostatic tissue.
(C)	Right Base:	Benign prostatic tissue.
(D)	Right Lat Apex:	Benign prostatic tissue.
(E)	Right Lat Mid:	Benign prostatic tissue.
(F)	Right Lat Base:	Benign prostatic tissue.
(G)	Left Apex:	Benign prostatic tissue. Immunostains for basal cell-specific high molecular weight keratin (34BE12), p63, racemase and c-myc support this diagnosis.
(H)	Left Mid:	Benign prostatic tissue.
(I)	Left Base:	Benign prostatic tissue. Immunostains for basal cell-specific high molecular weight keratin (34BE12), p63, racemase and c-myc support this diagnosis.
(J)	Left Lat Apex:	Benign prostatic tissue.
(K)	Left Lat Mid:	Benign prostatic tissue.
(L)	Left Lat Base:	Benign prostatic tissue.

4-28-09 (8:29 AM) no answer -KA
4-29-09 pt notified (?) J am having another pathologist review the case.

OK To Call pt.

Page 1 of 2

46

Pathology Report
Central Florida Urology Specialists

Central Florida Urology Specialists
Pathology Laboratory
1950 Laurel Manor Dr Bldg 210
The Villages, FL 32162

Accession number: **S09-00805**
Collected Date: 11 Jun 2009
Received Date: 11 Jun 2009
Report Date: 12 Jun 2009

Clinical: Prostate cancer.

Patient Information
Name: **Miller, Ira B**
DOB/SSN: ▓▓▓▓▓▓▓▓▓
Chart/Account#:

Referring Physician
Harvey Taub, M.D.
1950 Laurel Manor Dr Bldg 210
The Villages, FL 32162
352-430-0705   Fax: 352-430-0709

Base

10 Benign	7 Benign	1 Benign	4 CA, G6, 8%
11 Benign	8 Benign	2 CA, G6, 25%	5 Benign
12 Benign	9 Benign	3 Benign	6 Benign

L   R

Apex

#	Specimen Description	Pieces	Length (mm)	Blocks
1	Prostate Right Medial Base	1	16	1
2	Prostate Right Medial Mid	2	14-23	1
3	Prostate Right Medial Apex	2	16-21	1
4	Prostate Right Lateral Base	2	14-20	1
5	Prostate Right Lateral Mid	2	16-18	1
6	Prostate Right Lateral Apex	2	17-18	1
7	Prostate Left Medial Base	2	19-21	1
8	Prostate Left Medial Mid	2	18-22	1
9	Prostate Left Medial Apex	2	16-18	1
10	Prostate Left Lateral Base	2	8-20	1
11	Prostate Left Lateral Mid	2	13-13	1
12	Prostate Left Lateral Apex	2	13-14	1

CASE SUMMARY: Adenocarcinoma, Gleason score 6 (3+3). Tumor involves the right side of the prostate.

DIAGNOSIS:
(1) Prostate Right Medial Base: Benign prostate tissue.
(2) Prostate Right Medial Mid: Adenocarcinoma, Gleason score 6 (3+3), involving approximately 25% of the biopsy length.
(3) Prostate Right Medial Apex: Benign prostate tissue.
(4) Prostate Right Lateral Base: Adenocarcinoma, Gleason score 6 (3+3), involving approximately 8% of the biopsy length.
(5) Prostate Right Lateral Mid: Benign prostate tissue.
(6) Prostate Right Lateral Apex: Benign prostate tissue.
(7) Prostate Left Medial Base: Benign prostate tissue.
(8) Prostate Left Medial Mid: Benign prostate tissue.
(9) Prostate Left Medial Apex: Benign prostate tissue.
(10) Prostate Left Lateral Base: Benign prostate tissue.
(11) Prostate Left Lateral Mid: Benign prostate tissue.
(12) Prostate Left Lateral Apex: Benign prostate tissue.

William M Murphy, M.D., Pathologist
Electronically Signed (6/12/2009)

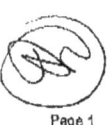

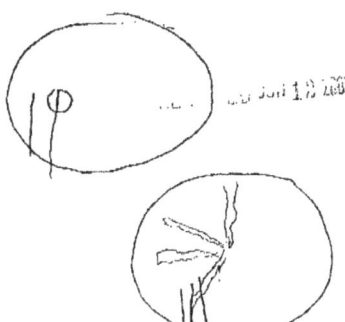

Page 1

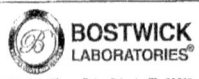

BOSTWICK LABORATORIES®

7001 Lake Ellenor Drive Orlando, FL 32809
Phone 407-888-9934   Fax 407-856-0333   www.bostwicklaboratories.com

SPECIMEN INFORMATION
Date Collected: 11/18/2010
Date Received: 11/19/2010
Date Reported: 11/22/2010 17:40

BL10-0102-0005199

PATIENT INFORMATION

Name:	Ira B Miller
SSN:	▮▮▮▮ Sex: Male
Date of Birth:	▮▮▮▮ Age: 55
Requisition # :	BU100164511 Chart #:
Phone:	▮▮▮▮

PHYSICIAN INFORMATION

Harvey C Taub M.D.
Associates for Urology Care
1901 SE 18th Ave
Building 300
Ocala, FL 34471

Phone: (352) 351-1313
Fax: (352) 351-1927

CLINICAL HISTORY

Provided ICD-9 codes: 790.93.

GROSS DESCRIPTION

PROSTATE, NEEDLE BIOPSIES:

The specimen was received in 12 vials containing pink-tan 0.1 cm diameter prostate biopsies in formalin; submitted in toto.

	Site	Length
(A1)	Right Apex	1.8, 1.1 cm (Bisected)
(B1)	Right Mid	2.0, 1.7 cm (Bisected, Fragmented)
(C1)	Right Base	2.0, 1.1 cm (Fragmented)
(D1)	Right Lat Apex	1.7, 1.6 cm (Fragmented)
(E1)	Right Lat Mid	2.0, 1.8 cm (Bisected, Fragmented, Stringy)
(F1)	Right Lat Base	2.1, 1.7 cm (Stringy, Fragmented)
(G1)	Left Apex	1.7, 1.7 cm (Stringy, Fragmented)
(H1)	Left Mid	1.4, 1.2 cm (Fragmented)
(I1)	Left Base	1.4, 1.2 cm
(J1)	Left Lat Apex	1.6, 1.5 cm (Fragmented)
(K1)	Left Lat Mid	2.1, 1.5 cm (Bisected, Fragmented, Stringy)
(L1)	Left Lat Base	1.3, 1.1 cm (Stringy, Fragmented)

*Biopsies submitted on blue sponge.

PROSTATE BIOPSY MAP

Left   Right

Base	BENIGN	BENIGN	BENIGN	BENIGN	Base
Mid	BENIGN	BENIGN	BENIGN	BENIGN	Mid
Apex	BENIGN	BENIGN	BENIGN	BENIGN	Apex

Lateral   Lateral

HGPIN ▨▨▨   SUSPICIOUS ▨▨▨   MALIGNANT ▨▨▨

DIAGNOSIS

PROSTATE, NEEDLE BIOPSIES:

(A1)	Right Apex:	Benign prostatic tissue.
(B1)	Right Mid:	Benign prostatic tissue.
(C1)	Right Base:	Benign prostatic tissue.
(D1)	Right Lat Apex:	Benign prostatic tissue.
(E1)	Right Lat Mid:	Benign prostatic tissue.
(F1)	Right Lat Base:	Benign prostatic tissue.
(G1)	Left Apex:	Benign prostatic tissue.
(H1)	Left Mid:	Benign prostatic tissue.
(I1)	Left Base:	Benign prostatic tissue.
(J1)	Left Lat Apex:	Benign prostatic tissue.
(K1)	Left Lat Mid:	Benign prostatic tissue.
(L1)	Left Lat Base:	Benign prostatic tissue.

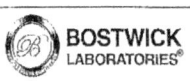

BOSTWICK LABORATORIES®

4851 Lake Brook Dr, Richmond, VA 23060

one 877-865-3262   Fax 804-545-9725   www.bostwicklaboratories.com

SPECIMEN INFORMATION

Date Collected: 11/18/2010 10:10
Date Received: 11/19/2010
Date Reported: 11/22/2010 12:28

CC10-0106-0070119

PATIENT INFORMATION

Name:	Ira B Miller	
SSN:		Sex: Male
Date of Birth:		Age: 55
Requisition #	BU100164528	Chart #:
Phone:		

PHYSICIAN INFORMATION

Harvey C Taub M.D.
Associates for Urology Care
1901 SE 18th Ave
Building 300
Ocala, FL 34471

Phone: (352) 351-1313
Fax: (352) 351-1927

CLINICAL HISTORY

Provided ICD-9 codes: 185. Received in Clinical Lab for testing on: 11/19/2010

TEST DESCRIPTIONS	TEST RESULTS		REFERENCE RANGE	LEGEND
Prostate Specific Antigen - Total	1.2	NORMAL	< 0.1 - 4.0 ng/ml	●

PATIENT TREND REPORT

2008	2009	2010

(graph showing values 1.3 Apr 2010 and 1.2 Nov 2010)

Previous Bx Diagnosis	May 2010 :Benign, Apr 2009 :Benign

NOTES:
- Some of the PSA values presented in the graph above may be provided by a laboratory independent of Bostwick Laboratories, Inc. and should not be construed as results derived by or from Bostwick Laboratories, Inc. testing. These values may have been obtained using different assay methods or kits and cannot be used interchangeably.

PSA TESTING
- Manufacturer: Siemens.
- Methodology: Automated Chemiluminescence System - Equimoisr Assay

Results cannot be interpreted as absolute evidence of the presence or absence of malignant disease.

William Glass, M.D., PhD., MBA

Page 1 of 1

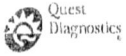
Quest
Diagnostics

Report Status: Final

MILLER, IRA B

Patient Information	Specimen Information	Client Information
MILLER, IRA B	Specimen: TM526723E Requisition: 0002724	Client #: ▓▓▓▓▓ 311.A999 KRAUCAK, NELSON
DOB: ▓▓▓▓ AGE: 54 Gender: M Phone: ▓▓▓▓▓ Patient ID: MI1955	Collected: 10/13/2010 / 08:10 EDT Received: 10/13/2010 / 23:22 EDT Reported: 10/20/2010 / 16:14 EDT (* A Copy Sent To)	LIFE FAMILY PRACTICE CENTER Attn: +++NEW 1501 N US HIGHWAY 441 STE 1702 THE VILLAGES, FL 32159-6802

Test Name	In Range	Out Of Range	Reference Range	Lab
LIPID PANEL				
CHOLESTEROL, TOTAL	146		125-200 mg/dL	TP
HDL CHOLESTEROL	44		> OR = 40 mg/dL	TP
TRIGLYCERIDES	51		<150 mg/dL	TP
LDL-CHOLESTEROL	92		<130 mg/dL (calc)	TP

Desirable range <100 mg/dL for patients with CHD or
diabetes and <70 mg/dL for diabetic patients with
known heart disease.

CHOL/HDLC RATIO	3.3		< OR = 5.0 (calc)	TP
PLEASE NOTE:				TP

We received your handwritten test order and
performed the AMA defined lipid panel. If
this is not what you intended to order, please
contact your local client service representative
immediately so that we may adjust our billing
appropriately. You may also inquire about
alternative or additional testing.

COMPREHENSIVE METABOLIC				TP
PANEL W/EGFR				
GLUCOSE	85		65-99 mg/dL	

Fasting reference interval

UREA NITROGEN (BUN)	24		7-25 mg/dL	
CREATININE	1.24		0.76-1.46 mg/dL	
eGFR NON-AFR. AMERICAN	>60		> OR = 60 mL/min/1.73m2	
eGFR AFRICAN AMERICAN	>60		> OR = 60 mL/min/1.73m2	
BUN/CREATININE RATIO	NOT APPLICABLE		6-22 (calc)	

Bun/Creatinine ratio is not reported when the BUN
and creatinine values are within normal limits.

SODIUM	141		135-146 mmol/L	
POTASSIUM	5.0		3.5-5.3 mmol/L	
CHLORIDE	106		98-110 mmol/L	
CARBON DIOXIDE	21		21-33 mmol/L	
CALCIUM	9.7		8.6-10.2 mg/dL	
PROTEIN, TOTAL	7.4		6.2-8.3 g/dL	
ALBUMIN	4.7		3.6-5.1 g/dL	
GLOBULIN	2.7		2.1-3.7 g/dL (calc)	
ALBUMIN/GLOBULIN RATIO	1.7		1.0-2.1 (calc)	
BILIRUBIN, TOTAL	0.5		0.2-1.2 mg/dL	
ALKALINE PHOSPHATASE	62		40-115 U/L	
AST	25		10-35 U/L	
ALT	18		9-60 U/L	
TSH, 3RD GENERATION	2.10		0.40-4.50 mIU/L	TP
T4 (THYROXINE), TOTAL	6.1		4.5-12.5 mcg/dL	TP
T3, TOTAL	93		76-181 ng/dL	TP
* DIHYDROTESTOSTERONE	56		25-75 ng/dL	AMD

CLIENT SERVICES: 866.697.8378   COLLECTED: 10/13/2010 08:10 EDT   PAGE 1 OF 2

Quest, Quest Diagnostics, the associated logo and all associated Quest Diagnostics marks are the trademarks of Quest Diagnostics.

50

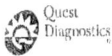

Quest
Diagnostics

Report Status: Final

MILLER, IRA B

Patient Information	Specimen Information	Client Information
MILLER, IRA B	Specimen: TM526723E	Client #: ▓▓▓▓
	Collected: 10/13/2010 / 08:10 EDT	KRAUCAK, NELSON
DOB: ▓▓▓▓ AGE: 54	Received: 10/13/2010 / 23:22 EDT	
Gender: M	Reported: 10/20/2010 / 16:14 EDT	
Patient ID: MI1955	(* A Copy Sent To)	

Test Name	In Range	Out Of Range	Reference Range	Lab
CBC (INCLUDES DIFF/PLT)				TP
WHITE BLOOD CELL COUNT	5.1		3.8-10.8 Thousand/uL	
RED BLOOD CELL COUNT	4.92		4.20-5.80 Million/uL	
HEMOGLOBIN	15.5		13.2-17.1 g/dL	
HEMATOCRIT	46.7		38.5-50.0 %	
MCV	94.9		80.0-100.0 fL	
MCH	31.6		27.0-33.0 pg	
MCHC	33.3		32.0-36.0 g/dL	
RDW	14.6		11.0-15.0 %	
PLATELET COUNT	228		140-400 Thousand/uL	
ABSOLUTE NEUTROPHILS	3009		1500-7800 cells/uL	
ABSOLUTE LYMPHOCYTES	1372		850-3900 cells/uL	
ABSOLUTE MONOCYTES	408		200-950 cells/uL	
ABSOLUTE EOSINOPHILS	270		15-500 cells/uL	
ABSOLUTE BASOPHILS	41		0-200 cells/uL	
NEUTROPHILS	59.0		%	
LYMPHOCYTES	26.9		%	
MONOCYTES	8.0		%	
EOSINOPHILS	5.3		%	
BASOPHILS	0.8		%	
DHEA SULFATE	155		25-240 mcg/dL	TP
TESTOSTERONE, FREE AND				AMD
TOTAL, LC/MS/MS				
TESTOSTERONE, TOTAL	655		250-1100 ng/dL	
TESTOSTERONE, FREE				
PERCENT		2.39 H	1.50-2.20 %	
FREE TESTOSTERONE		156.5 H	35.0-155.0 pg/mL	

PERFORMING SITE:

AMD   QUEST DIAGNOSTICS/CHANTILLY, 14225 NEWBROOK DRIVE, CHANTILLY, VA 20151-2228 Laboratory Director: KENNETH L. SISCO, MD, CLIA: 49D0221801
TP   QUEST DIAGNOSTICS-TAMPA, 4225 E. FOWLER AVE, TAMPA, FL 33617 Laboratory Director: LUIS A DIAZ-ROSARIO,MD, CLIA: 10D0291120

* Copy To Client: AVECILLA,GUILLERMO B MD

[handwritten notes]

CLIENT SERVICES: 866.697.8378   COLLECTED: 10/13/2010 08:10 EDT   PAGE 2 OF 2

Quest, Quest Diagnostics, the associated logo and all associated Quest Diagnostics marks are the trademarks of Quest Diagnostics.

51

Chapter 5

GETTING STARTED

Cleansing

Why did we get cancer in the first place? That is something that you and I may never know, although, I have my suspicions like what I mentioned in the last chapter. Did hard living, drinking and partying have something to do with this for me? Did my younger life as a beach bum surfer dude and overexposure to the sun have something to do with this? We didn't know what sun screen was when I was growing up. Actually, everyone put on suntan *oil* to *INCREASE* the sun exposure, not deter it. Or, was it something in the water….?

It is my opinion that there was something within my body that caused this cancer. How was I going to get rid of it and how was I going to make sure that it doesn't come back and I never have to face this again? What I do know today is that my body was out of balance with where it should be. I also have my suspicions about the tap water that I drank and bathed in all my life. With so many toxins in the ground water today, as I lived on well water for a long period of time in my life and with so many chemicals going into purifying city water, I think that this could have had a cause as well. Not only that but I just recently moved into a brand new home and maybe the new CPVC plumbing had something to do with it. For more in-depth information on water go to a link online: http://www.healingdaily.com/detoxification-diet/water-filtration-systems.htm)

So, the first thing that I did when I learned that I had cancer was to go through an intensive internal cleansing program and detoxify my body. I had tried colon cleansing twice before when I was seeking ways to help improve my stamina and mental awareness and consequently learned about my low levels of testosterone. I had heard through commercials and internet searching about the effects of a clogged colon. I went out and bought another cleansing kit and the one that I bought was called, "**Men's Rebuild**" by Yerba Prima.

Some of the things that I learned online were about all the gross things that you can expect to come out of your body once you started the cleansing process. If you go online there are actual pictures of some of the things that come out of your body in your stool. I couldn't believe some of the things that I saw but when I did this myself and upon examination of my own stool, it was true what I was seeing. Not to get too repulsive but it is amazing some of the things that are clogging up your colon. Long white stringy things and black tar ball looking things come out of you that you would never think is normal to come out of anyone. So, there are things that are inside you that need not be there.

Your colon is not like a smooth pipe inside where waste would smoothly pass through. It has pockets that tend to trap things inside. It is an internal sewer system and tends to get clogged up with this sludge that you have to clean out from time to time. However, I must warn you. There are poisons trapped in your colon, in these pockets, and as you cleanse you release these poisons back into your body and there are some ill effects that will be felt when these toxins are released. You will feel like you have the flu or that you have been poisoned. This lasted for 4 days for me the first time that I did the cleansing process. I was sooo tempted to stop cleansing as I thought that it was the product that was making me sick but soon learned that it was the poisons coming out of my body that was doing this. To be quite honest, it was another year before I attempted cleansing again because of the apprehension of these ill effects. And sure enough, when I did it again the same thing happened but it was not for the duration that it was the first time. This time these ill effects only lasted 3 days and the third day was not too bad. It did make me realize that I didn't want to go long periods of time any more to cleanse. I didn't want to have to go through the extreme effects that it had on me the first time that I cleansed and hopefully any other subsequence times I would see less and less ill effects in the beginning.

An unexpected result did happen from my cleansing the first time and this really told me that colon cleansing was not just a health freaks fairytale. Some people may be skeptical and say that colon cleansing is crazy or fanatical but I assure you that it is not. This was proven to me in the release of the poisons in my body that gave me those ill effects but it also made me a believer when after I went through the cleansing process my sweat was not wretched like it had been for years.

I study martial arts and while I was taking a form of martial arts known as Juko Kai I would come home with

54

my karate gi (uniform) soaked with sweat and it had a really wretched sour smell to it. My gi was actually a heavy judo style gi. A judo gi is especially heavy so your opponent can grab you by your gi and throw you without the gi tearing or ripping. But this heavy gi also made me sweat profusely. When I would come home, my wife Patti would immediately throw it into the washer because it smelled so bad and heaven forbid it sat in the hamper for days. She would even wash it separately because she feared that my stench might come out into the other clothes in the wash. But after my first colon cleansing which lasted for 21 days an amazing thing happened. I asked, "Honey, does my gi stink as much as it used to"? She said, "No, not anything like it used to". Wow... I was blown away by this. And I have not had a stench about me like that ever since.

So, I am a true believer that colon cleansing works. It is imperative that you rid these poisons and toxins from your body. If not then there is a good chance that your cancer will return or a new form of cancer will attack your body. There is no telling how many years that I carried these impurities around in my body and I absolutely believe that this had something to do with my prostate and skin cancer. Not only that but I would bet that it had something to do with my acid reflux as well. So once I learned that I had prostate cancer I immediately went out and bought a colon cleansing kit and started my program. And that is what it is too. It is a program that you are on from 16 to 30 days depending on how much cleansing you want to do for your body. This time I did it for the full 30 days. And trust me, it is not easy to be on and stay on this program. It takes a lot of discipline, as does this whole entire program that I am writing this book about. This whole cancer fighting program takes a lot of discipline and you must put yourself on a strict schedule, but it is well worth the results. So just have the mindset that you are in it for the long haul. But it's worth it because you cannot put a price on your life or your health. I did the colon cleansing again 6 months later too. I wanted to make sure that I got all the impurities out of my system and I will, from now on, make sure that I cleanse my colon every six months. And in case you are wondering, yes I had the ill feeling and light headedness when I again did the colon cleansing once I learned I had prostate cancer. But, the second one in 6 months was only a mild case for a day or day and a half. That alone will make me want to continue to do this every six months. And there is some good news that I can report. The last time that I cleansed I had no ill effects at all.

Another thing that colon cleansing does is it allows your now clean colon to absorb the maximum amount of nutrients from the food, herbs and supplements that you take. I wanted to make sure that I had maximum absorption of any cancer treating herbs and supplements that I was getting ready to take to combat this cancer. This was war. I wanted all the benefits that I could possibly derive from what I was about to do and undertake. And colon cleansing every six months was going to assure this for me. A byproduct of colon cleansing is that this enhances your immune system as well. I used to get sick two or three times a year. I have yet to get sick this year. It also helps in fighting the aging process. Think about it. If you never cleansed your colon, then the buildup on the walls of your colon will cause a decrease in nutrient absorption as you age and your body will be starved of the much needed nutrients to keep you feeling young and alive.

Something else that you have to do is take Bentonite. Bentonite is made from volcanic clay and it removes heavy metals from your body. I use "Sonne's 7" and "Great Plains Bentonite". Great Plaines Bentonite is already in the **Men's Renew** but I took the Sonne's 7 for added measures. It is my belief, as well as a lot of others, that heavy metals in your body can and are the cause of cancer in your body. So for me it was imperative to cleanse any heavy metals out of my body that I might have. There are kits for testing heavy metals in your body that I soon learned of but not in time before I started my program. I just went and did the program to remove any heavy metals that I may have had. Now I wish that I had taken this test so I would have known if I did have a lot of heavy metals in my body. Go to www.evenbetternow.com and learn more for yourself about heavy metal contamination of your body and take the test yourself.

I suspect that underarm deodorant alone can contribute to heavy metal toxicity. It contains aluminum and anything that you put on your body your skin will absorb. I remember one time I found a small hole around my bath tub where ants were going in and out of the base board. I took some concentrated liquid Sevin insect poison and dripped a little around the base board and then I took my finger and spread it around. Oh, was that a mistake. I had just poisoned myself and I was so sick I had to go see the doctor the next day. He gave me some belladonna pills which are an anti-poison prescription. So the lesson here is never put anything on your skin that you don't want inside your body and it is so easy to get things into your body that you don't want there and you need to remove. Another source of heavy metal poisoning can be fillings in your teeth, smoking, and even fumes from automobile exhaust can cause you to absorb heavy metals into your body. Also, there are a lot of things in your water, whether you have city water or well water that you would never know is there that you may not want in your body.

I didn't notice any physical affects from taking Bentonite like I did with the colon cleansing and I didn't notice any benefit from it either. However, I will bet there were a lot of benefits that I attained from taking it. Like I said, I just wish that I took a heavy metal test just to know. I don't know if it is a coincidence but 2 years after I moved into my new home, from a home where I had well water, I was diagnosed with prostate cancer AND my German Shepherd was diagnosed with cancer as well. I had to put her to sleep a month after she was diagnosed. She was too far gone for me to help her and it really saddened me to know what I know now and was not able to get her diagnosed in time to save her. The scary thing is that even my neighbor's dog passed away, I learned, about a month before mine did. So, I do not trust the water that I have at my house and we now drink bottled water although there are risks to that as well. The best source of water is through a filtration system in your home. Again, see the internet link above to learn all about this. I would highly recommend that you have your drinking water source tested to see what kind of chlorine and contaminates may be in it. The third cleansing agent that I have to tell you about is called Essiac Tea. A good website to go to learn about this natural miracle is http://www.healthfreedom. info/Cancer%20Essiac.htm. The trade name or brand that I use is called Flor-Essence.

You can buy it either in a bottle ready to go or you can buy the herbs and brew your own. I preferred to brew my own as it was stronger, fresher and was less expensive this way. Essiac tea is no longer touted as an anti-cancer product as it once was but as a detoxifier of the body. In any case, I immediately got on the Essiac tea program and have stayed on it to keep my body detoxified during this whole process and cleansing at the cellular level.

The definition of cancer is: any malignant growth or tumor caused by abnormal and uncontrolled *cell* division (wordnetweb.princeton.edu/perl/webwn) -*It has been rightly said that both health and disease begin in the cells, for it is at the cellular level that the vast majority of the body's multitude of interactions occur* (page 3 The Acid/Alkaline Food Guide) Drinking Essiac tea will detoxify your body and get your body healing at the cellular level since cancer is a disease of the cells. I was attacking cancer at its core, healing abnormal cells and keeping the normal cells healthy and growing in place of the abnormal ones. Essiac Tea is essential to this program.

So now I cleansed my colon of poisons and toxins that were trapped in my colon, I cleansed the heavy metals out of my body and lastly I am detoxifying my body and cleansing at the cellular level. I was ready to go. Now that I took all the bad things out of my body I was ready to put nothing but good things back in. (One side note: At this time I am studying up on parasites within your body. While that may not be a cause of cancer it may be something that you would want to check out in your cleansing process. You might as well get everything out and your insides cleaned... I would Google body parasites and read up on that. You will not believe what you will find out and see in pictures there.)

IMPORTANT NOTE: One important supplement to put back in after cleansing is a good probiotic. When you cleanse you are basically cleaning everything out of your digestive system including the *good* bacterium that keeps your immune system strong. Probiotics quickly put the good bacteria back into your colon to keep your immune system strong and healthy. I use Dr. Ohhira's Professional Grade. A strong immune system is very important in the battle against cancer. We will learn all about that in detail in the Herbs and Supplements chapter.

Chapter 6

<u>DIET</u>

When I went to Mayo in October of '08 one of the tests that they did was a fat content test. They sit you in this space capsule looking contraption and the technician puts pressurized air into the capsule to determine what percentage body fat you have. I was shocked at what I learned. I thought that I was in great shape but I was stunned to learn that I had 23% body fat. That was termed as having "Excess Fat" in your body. As a by-product of my regimen to cure my cancer, I came up with what I needed to do to change my diet and as an unexpected result lost this body fat. The first thing that I did was make a radical change in what I put in my mouth and my body. This is a "life change" not just a change in my diet. You really have to accept that the food that you have been eating is the same thing that is possibly killing you. I lost 20 pounds in the first three months that I was on this life style diet. I went from 195 pounds to 175 pounds. The funny thing was that people thought that my losing this weight was due to the cancer and thought that I looked emaciated and "sunken in"; that I looked sick, like a real cancer patient. People were worried and said that I needed to gain weight. I just laughed and said that I lost the weight on purpose and it was an after-effect of my change in eating habits. I dropped a full waist size from a size 33 to a size 32. Even though I had 23% body fat content I was still not all that big to begin with like you see in a lot of over-weigh guys. So there wasn't really much to lose in my waist. If I was a size 42 or something like that, or more, then there would have been a lot more to lose. So going from a size 33 to a size 32 was actually a big deal for me. If you are more overweight then chances are you will see a greater result than what I did.

I was a chocoholic, too. I love chocolate. Hershey's Semi-sweet chocolate was my favorite. Just writing about it to this day makes me want to go out and get some. Do you know how there are just some things in life that when you cut them out of your life you never lose that craving for? I know that cigarettes are another thing people crave. Just ask those folks who quit. But I was and still am a real sucker for sweets. I think that out of everything, cutting out the sweets has been the toughest challenge for me. It seems that my body just craves things that are sweet like cookies, cakes, ice cream, and all things chocolate. But as you will see below, sugar is one of the deadliest foods for a cancer victim.

Red meat was another thing that I cut out of my diet. Who doesn't love a nice thick rib-eye grilled to perfection on the grill? Mmmm Mmmm Well, my wife Patti doesn't but she's weird anyway. But I learned that burnt flesh is very carcinogenic and when you get those burnt stripes on the steak as you grill it it is really causing that meat to become carcinogenic. In Prevention Magazine (October 2010 pg. 36) it says *Processed, charred and well-done meats can contain cancer causing heterocyclic amines, which form when meat is seared at high temperatures and polycyclic aromatic hydrocarbons, which get into food when it is charcoal broiled.* They go on to say that to counteract this phenomenon you should add rosemary and thyme to your marinade to cut down on up to 87% of the carcinogenic

HCA's. Bacon is another one. It is extremely carcinogenic and the more you cook it the worse it gets. So I just cut out beef and pork all together and I only ate chicken.

The best chicken to get is organic chicken and the "Free Range" organic chicken if you can find it. It is usually very hard to find though. I usually settled on the organic chicken. This is the chicken that is absent of hormones, preservatives and pesticides. It usually says on the package that they are only grain fed also. The reason Free Range chickens are so good for you is because they are allowed to roam around the farm and are not kept in cages. This is better because caged chickens are likely to eat their own feces if they are locked up in a cage 24/7. I was really surprised when I read an article in Men's Fitness magazine (September 2008 pg. 92) and it said not to waste your money on buying organic chicken. I think that someone forgot to do their homework on this one. In the article it also said that it agreed that conventional wisdom held that pesticides are bad for our health even though the federal government has yet to come up with some guidelines on what is acceptable in pesticides in or on our foods and what is not acceptable. The term "Organic" says that the product is deemed pesticide free as well as hormone free. So how can they say not to waste your money on buying organic chicken? It didn't make sense.

Organic eggs are better as well and again, free range chicken eggs are best for the same reasons that I mentioned above. I eat a lot of eggs and especially raw ones in my protein shakes that I make at least twice a day. You have to be careful of raw eggs though. I had eaten some raw ones years ago that were infected with salmonella (or so I suspected) and oh man did they make me sick. I felt like I was ready to die. I *wanted* to die I was so sick. The last time that happened I swore off raw eggs for about 2 years. I am currently back on raw eggs, though. I guess I am a glutton for punishment. They really are a good source of protein. I like to mix up my protein sources. But, today, you can get pasteurized eggs and this will take out the worry or possibility of you getting salmonella.

Whey protein is the best source of protein for just waking up in the morning and for an after-workout shake. This protein is great for a fast assimilation of protein to build and repair muscles. However, I feel that putting some egg, milk and even some yogurt in there is a good mixture and assimilates well in your body. It makes for a thick tasty shake too. Another thing that I like to put in my protein shakes are *frozen* fruits; bananas, mixed fruit and blueberries. You can find the mixed fruit and blueberries in a bag in your grocer's freezer department. Blueberries are a great antioxidant and cancer fighter. I found that when your bananas start getting too ripe the best thing to do is peel them and put them in a freezer bag and freeze them. This really makes for a nice cold thick shake. Naturally sweetens the shake as well. What I have learned is to make a double batch of protein shake which consists of 2 eggs, 8 ounces of water, 4 ounces of milk, 4 ounces of almond milk and some frozen fruit to taste. Then, while you are mixing this up in the blender throw in 2 heaping scoops of protein with some wheat grass. I also put in a tablespoon of psyllium husks to keep my colon healthy and working properly with waste removal. I drink half before I go to work out and then the other half when I get back (within a half hour of getting back). I work out in the mornings so this is part of my breakfast. If you work out in the evenings it would be the opposite for you. Also in the evening, right before bed, I drink a shake with casein protein as this doesn't assimilate in your body as fast as whey. It slowly releases the protein amino acids as you sleep over a longer period of time and this helps in getting the necessary nutrients into your body and helps to repair your body as well. This is very necessary when fighting off cancer.

And speaking of sleep, sleep is extremely important as well. You HAVE to get your proper amount of sleep as, again, this allows the repair process to take place in your body and this is where the good cells take over the bad cancer cells that are dying from the process that I am describing in this book. I would suggest that you get a minimum of 8 hours sleep. If you work this program like I have described and have kids like I do, you will find this difficult to do. But no matter what it takes, you have to get the sleep you need to rebuild yourself from the attack of the cancer. I had to go to my managers at work and I explained to them that it takes a while in the morning for me to get through my routine and that I need my sleep. They understood to a point, however, what I was doing was never heard of so they were skeptical to say the least. I would hope that any understanding boss would understand it if you lay out your whole routine to them. You may even have to give this book to them to read to understand what you are doing.

My routine was to get up in the morning, take my IP6 w/ Inositol first thing on an empty stomach, make my shake and drink half of the protein shake. Then I would make my Budwig recipe, heat my purified water for the Essiac tea and then eat the Budwig Recipe and drink the tea together. After that I would go work out, come back, drink the other half of my shake, take a shower and then take my supplements with CELLFOOD mixed in purified water as I was headed out the door. All this meant that I needed to wake up at 6 am so I could be at work by 10 am. Then I would do it all again at night. I would come home, drink the IP6 w/ Inositol first thing on an empty stomach when I got in the door, then I made my Budwig Recipe. The Essiac tea I would make mid-evening after dinner after my food settled. Then before bed I took my supplements and another protein shake. Protein has amino acids in it, as I mentioned earlier, that are essential building blocks for building muscle but also for the repair of anything that is in need of repair in your body…like cancer. That was my daily routine. That meant that you had to be in bed by 10 pm to get the proper sleep and rest so that repairs could take place.

Another thing that I did was swear off fried foods. Nothing fried includes potato chips, french fries, fried chicken etc. This, too, was extremely hard to do. Not only did I narrow down my meat of choice to only organic chicken, now I eliminated half the ways to cook chicken. And boy do I love fried chicken wings. There is a little diner in Wildwood called The Old Coffee House where they have the best fried chicken in the world. Nine months into my diet plan I broke down and hit The Old Coffee House and pigged out. I couldn't help it and chances are you won't be able to either. I was really good for about the first 6 months. I not only wanted to get myself better but I had a book to write and something to prove to the world. Now, with the recent good results, I eased up and I would eat fried chicken wings now and then … and once in a great while I will go visit The Old Coffee House. However, I did perfect *grilled* chicken wings on the bar-b-que grill. I have had some rave reviews on these and people tell me that they are better than the fried ones. You'll have to e-mail me though if you want the recipe.

I mentioned above that I fell off the fried chicken wagon but I do not advocate cheating on your diet. I am, however, a realist. Look at it this way; you are doing this to cure yourself of a deadly disease, keeping yourself from having surgery, not wanting to mess up what you did for your colon cleansing, lose weight and look fantastic. It is such a pleasure when people come up to me and tell me how great that I look 25 pounds lighter. I am always quick to share with them how I did it. I am really excited to be able to go back to Mayo and get in that body fat machine and see what the results are there. But where I was going with this, the longer you stay on the diet the better off you will be and the faster your results will be as well. I wish now that I had stayed on my diet as I would have gotten healthy and cured the cancer just that much faster.

Basically, my whole diet looked like this: Budwig and protein shake in the morning, a fresh salad with cottage cheese in the afternoon and then chicken with a potato or rice and a fresh vegetable in the evening. All I drank was water with lemon too. I cut out all sodas and sweet tea. Now and then I would drink plain un-sweet tea with no sweeteners. I feel even those sugar alternatives are bad for you and maybe even worse. Just read the warning on the packet. I had to get really creative with cooking chicken. Mostly it was baked chicken breast but every now and then I would slice a chicken breast in two and fry it in a pan with olive oil. I don't mean cut it in half. I mean to slice it through the middle and make two thin halves and fry them up. I know that I said that I cut out all fried foods but you can only cook and eat baked chicken so many ways. So this was a nice alternative. I feel that olive oil is not that bad as a cooking source and I ate it with all my salads along with balsamic vinegar every day too. Olive oil is what I used on my chicken wings that I barbequed. If you do some research, you will find that people in Italy have a low rate of heart disease and they contribute this to them using a lot of olive oil in and on their foods. So I reasoned that it really can't be that bad for you. As a result, I am cured of cancer so there must be something to olive oil. The fried foods that I was mostly referring to would be those fried foods that you would get at restaurants. There they would fry foods in oil that has trans-fats in them, has been heated to temperatures that would break down these oils and cause them to become carcinogenic and be in these fryers for many hours if not days. This is a far cry from using fresh, cold pressed olive oil to cook with.

My potatoes would be mostly sweet potatoes because I didn't want to eat just a plain dry russet or baked potato. I wanted to put as little fat in my diet as I could so I didn't want to use any butter if I could avoid it. I don't use butter at all anyway. I use Smart Balance Butter Spread with the Extra Virgin Olive Oil; no trans-fats. On occasion we would have mashed potatoes and you can't make mashed potatoes without butter and milk so we would use the Smart Balance for that.

I ate a lot of broccoli too. I ate it raw and I ate it cooked. Since I was taking OncoPlex, that was a derivative of broccoli, I figured that I needed to add broccoli as a food as well. I would use fresh broccoli whenever I could, in my salads as well as steamed for dinner. I read somewhere that people should eat "live" things like fruits and vegetables rather than dead things like meat. Meat supposedly just rots in your digestive system since it takes so long to digest where fruits and vegetables are digested a lot easier. So that is why I swore off read meat and only ate organic chicken. Organic chicken was the lesser of the evils of meat. Personally, I couldn't just live off of fruits and vegetables. I need some meat in my diet. I did discover canned organic chicken in the grocery store and ate that on occasion to salads for lunch. Looking back, I don't know if that was such a good idea as it had to have preservatives in it if it came in a can but I needed to break up the monotony of only salads for lunch, on occasion.

Fruits I would eat a lot of as they were a good alternative to sweets that I cut out of my diet. I would eat fruit as an in-between meals snack. This healthy diet didn't seem to be very filling so the fruits came in very handy. Different vegetables were good for dinner as they broke up the monotony of chicken and potatoes. I tried to eat just fresh vegetables and nothing canned or frozen. I didn't want the preservatives that came in canned or some frozen foods.

I also introduced fresh tomatoes into my diet. I am someone who does not like vegetables that are in the "night shade" family. This includes tomatoes and onions. But I was taking Lycopene for my prostate which is a derivative of tomatoes so I figured that I better eat fresh tomatoes as well. This went along with the same thinking about the broccoli. So with every salad I had some cherry tomatoes.

Lastly, and probably most important of all is sugar. In investigating causes and cures for cancer I discovered that sugar is a demon, a real killer. **Sugar fuels cancer cells.** Let me repeat that a little louder...**SUGAR FUELS CANCER CELLS!** It is what cancer feeds on. The saying "Sugar feeds cancer" is simple. The explanation is a little more involved. Of the over 4 million cancer patients being treated in the U.S. today, almost none are offered any scientifically guided nutritional therapy other than being told to "just eat good foods." Many cancer patients would have a major improvement in their conditions if they controlled the supply of cancer's preferred fuel: GLUCOSE. Our body's primary source of energy takes the form of glucose. This type of simple sugar comes from digesting carbohydrates into a chemical that we can easily convert to energy. Keeping glucose within a normal range is extremely important to health and controlling your cancers growth. By slowing cancer's growth patients make it possible for their immune systems to catch up to the disease. Controlling one's blood-glucose levels through diet (little or no sugar), exercise, supplements, meditation and limiting prescription drugs - when necessary - can be one of the most crucial components to a cancer treatment program. The sad truth is, there is sugar added to just about everything in the first place. Look at the ingredients in the foods that you buy. Look at all the sugar that is in all these food items. It is ridiculous. So to go out and eat candy, ice cream, cookies, cakes, donuts, soda and/or even sweet tea (which I drank by the gallons) on top of all the other foods that you eat that has *hidden* sugar in it is insane when you have cancer. Don't do it. Swear off the intentional sugars at least until you have cured your cancer. I would never advocate going back to ingesting processed sugar ever again, but as I have said before, I am a realist and I know that we are only human and will want that occasional candy bar, or cookie or piece of cake at a birthday party. If you must you must but don't make it a habit. Today, I still only drink water with lemon. Just think of all the sugars and empty calories that you eliminate by merely drinking only water and the lemon helps burn calories. Do whatever it takes to defeat this scourge called cancer.

German scientist, Otto Warburg, Ph.D., the 1931 Nobel laureate in medicine, first discovered that cancer cells have a fundamentally different energy metabolism compared to healthy cells. The gist of his Nobel thesis was this, and I quote: malignant tumors frequently exhibit an increase in "anaerobic glycolysis" - a process whereby glucose is used by cancer cells as a fuel with lactic acid as an anaerobic by-product - compared to normal tissues. The large amount of lactic acid produced by this fermentation of glucose from the cancer cells is then transported to the liver. This conversion of glucose to lactate creates a lower, more acidic pH in cancerous tissues as well as overall physical fatigue from lactic acid build-up. Therefore, larger tumors tend to exhibit a more acidic pH.

Sugar also suppresses your immune system which I have said is so important in curing cancer. You need a strong immune system when combating cancer. Sugar raises the insulin level, which inhibits the release of growth hormones, which in turn depresses the immune system. (www.healingdaily.com) So, I cut out all sugars. This was not easy as I have mentioned. Go to www.healingdaily.com/detoxification-diet/sugar.htm. This will give you more of the technical aspects of why you want to cut out allllll sugar.

PUTTING YOUR BODY INTO THE PROPER ALKALINE STATE

As mentioned, tumors are very acidic due to the fermentation process of glucose to lactic acid by cancer cells. This in turn tends to make your whole body reside in a more acidic state as well. That is why you want to test yourself with pH test strips and see what state your body is in. You want your body to be in its proper pH balance. Ideally, you want your body to be in a pH balance of around 7.4, slightly alkaline. Below 7 your body gets into a more acidic state and there the cancer will thrive in an acidic body. It cannot thrive in an alkaline body so you want to get your body into an alkaline state.

All forms of arthritis are associated with excess acidity as well. In an acid state the acid erodes the calcium in the bones. Whatever health situation you are faced with, you can monitor your progress toward a proper acid/alkaline balance by testing your saliva pH. When healthy, the pH of blood is 7.4, the pH of spinal fluid is 7.4, and the pH of saliva is 7.4. Thus the pH of saliva parallels the extra cellular fluid and represents the most consistent and most definitive physical sign of the ionic calcium deficiency syndrome. The pH of the non-deficient and healthy person is in the 7.5 to 7.1 slightly alkaline range. The range from 6.5 which is weakly acidic to 4.5 which is strongly acidic represents states from mildly deficient to strongly deficient, respectively. Most children are a pH of 7.5. Over half of adults are a pH of 6.5 or lower, reflecting the calcium deficiency of aging and lifestyle defects. Cancer patients are usually a pH of 4.5, especially when terminal. You may want to get and read the book *The Calcium Factor: The Scientific Secret of Health and Youth*, by Robert R. Barefoot and Carl J. Reich. There is a lot of good information that backs up what I am saying here and backs up what this website, where I obtained all this information, is saying. Another great book that you need to get is "The Acid-Alkaline Food Guide" to know what foods to eat to keep your body in an alkaline state. It also goes into why you want your body in an alkaline state as well as how to get it there.

The website that I found all this information on is from an internet site at: www.healingdaily.com/ conditions/ saliva-ph-test.htm You can also find out where to order pH test strips here on this website to see if your body is currently in a pH balanced state. I got mine at Amazon.com, though. I wish that I would have done this before I started this program. But, I didn't know about any of this before I started. You have a unique advantage over me because you are getting all the right information up front and all at once.

So the bottom line is, sugar suppresses the immune system and feeds cancer which in turn causes your pH balance to go from an alkaline state to an acidic state which is the state that cancer thrives in. Remember, we want to starve and kill the cancer at its cellular level and replace it with healthy cells. So, stay away from sugars as much as possible and put your body in an alkaline pH state by eating the right foods. Taking apple cider vinegar everyday helps put you in an alkaline state, too. There is more about acid vs. alkalinity in Chapter 8.

Epilogue:
I went back to Mayo and my body fat was down to 15%. The girl who performed the test said that was very good. I was so happy. Hmm, I wonder where I would have been had I not been cheating?

Chapter 7

EXERCISE

Exercise….. I knew that part of my routine had to be exercise. One of the biggest problems that I always had was hurting my shoulder in the past and having to quit exercising to let it heal and then invariably I would get out of the routine of exercise and not go back for years…. This happened to me my whole life. I would get back into weight lifting, which I loved to do the most (my vanity I guess) and without fail it would happen again and again; my shoulders would give out and I would get out of my routine again and not go back for a year or years. Finally, just recently, I ran into a guy named Michael at the gym. He was wearing a bandage around his shoulder and I said "What happened to you?" He told me that he just had surgery to repair a torn rotator cuff muscle and he told me about all the pain that he was having. At that time my pain was just starting to come back to my shoulder because it always seemed that just when I started to get up there over the 155 pound flat bench press mark (I know, all you gym rats, that's not a lot of weight-Quit laughing) my shoulder would start hurting me. Then I would have to back down off the heavy weight… again. It got so bad this last time that I had to get off bench pressing with the bar totally and only use 30 pound dumbbells.

I saw Michael about 3 weeks later and he was on the cable machine doing these exercises where he would hold his arms down to his side and then at the elbow bring his hand and forearm up perpendicular to the upper part of his arm. He would take the handle that was attached to the cable machine and bring his hand across the front of his body with the handle pulling from both sides of your body. He would start out with doing one arm and pulling the handle from the inside of your body to the outside and then switch arms and go from the outside of your body pulling the handle across to the inside. Then he turned around and did the opposite arm. He only used the lightest weight that the machine had to offer. He did three sets of 15 repetitions with each arm. He suggested that I do this to help me with my problem. I was so desperate that I would try anything. As I did these exercises my shoulders seemed a lot stronger and I have not had any of the problems I was having. Today I am pushing 225 pounds and no pain in my shoulders. See, I told you there is a lot of information in this book other than just about cancer.

You will come up with your own workout routine. I prefer to use weights and machines to give my body strength and definition. I also was taking karate 3 nights a week. That was a great cardio workout. I cannot think of a better cardio program than karate. Not only are you exercising but you are learning self-defense and stretching your muscles for better mobility and flexibility. What can be better than that? But if you are not into weight lifting and/or karate then come up with your own routines that you like. It has to be something that you LOVE to do so you will stay with it. You can run, play tennis, do the cardio machines at the gym, anything to get your heart rate up and sustain it for a period of time to get the aerobic benefits from exercise. Very important! By getting your heart rate up you are getting your breathing up and by getting your breathing up you are oxygenating your body. You are also getting your blood pumping which is getting all the needed nutrients to your body and to the cells in your body quicker, which in turn helps you heal and cure yourself more rapidly.

With working out should come massages, whirlpools, saunas and steam baths for relaxation. Relaxation is very important to reducing stress. Stress is very harmful to your health. The job that I was in when I was diagnosed with cancer had me under a tremendous amount of stress. Every day I would go to work wondering if I was going to be fired because of the demands that the executive management team put on the employees there. I am an independent, out of the box thinker and where I worked they didn't like someone like me. They just wanted someone that they can give rules to and tell them to do it or else. It was terrible. I loved my career; I just didn't like all the stress that the company I was working for put me under. Even one of the Executive Managers would joke (but maybe not so much of a joke in reality) that he would drive to work with his fingers crossed on the steering wheel of his car hoping that he still had a job there that day. I think that a large part of me getting cancer was due to all this stress. Today, I have changed jobs. I am working for an independent real estate firm and I love it. The only stress that I have now is the stress that I put on myself to succeed. I have been working there for 2 years now and I attribute part of the cure of my cancer to getting away from all the stress that I was under at my old job. When I first left my old company I was traumatized because I didn't like change and I had a routine built up there (even though I was miserable there). But now, 2 years later, I look back and I see what a blessing it really was. I am extremely successful now in my new job. I love it so much more even though I am not making as much money. I was recognized with a letter of accommodation from the CEO of ERA Real Estate and a certificate all in my first year there. So don't be afraid of change. Life is too short to stay somewhere where you are miserable and under a lot of stress.

I thought about taking yoga too. I think that would be awesome. To date I have not come across any yoga facilities that are convenient for me. If any of you have experienced positive effects from yoga I would love to hear from you. I did go on a cruise recently and decided that my wife and I would take the yoga class that they were giving on the private island that they were stopping at. We took this hour long class and to my amazement, my knees that were hurting no longer were hurting me. "Wow... I may be on to something here." Thinking back to just a year ago when I was taking karate my knees didn't hurt then and that probably was attributed to all the stretching and kicking that I did. This kicking I think, kept my legs strong and the stretching helped as well. So when I took yoga on the beach and we did all this stretching and calisthenics, it helped my knees a lot. Now I make sure that I work out my lower body (I never used to do that, it was all upper body) and do some stretching too. I would recommend that anyone with sore knees do this before considering having surgery. Get on a good leg workout routine. Have a professional make up a workout for you to hit all the muscles of your legs.

One time I hurt my left knee from jogging and then right after jogging kicking a soccer ball with my son. I guess that by running I weakened the supporting muscles in my knees and I ended up tearing my meniscus when I kicked the soccer ball with the side of my foot so much. This knee got so bad that I had to have a shot of cortisone. But before I did I walked around in pain for 2 weeks. In those 2 weeks I went up to North Carolina to go skiing and couldn't even ski, my knee hurt so much. When I got back I went straight to the doctor and made an appointment. But in the mean time I favored my left leg so much that my right knee began to hurt. Now both knees were hurting. I thought, "I guess that just comes with old age". But this yoga came along and then I started working out my legs on the machines at the YMCA. Now my knees feel fine. I highly recommend that you just use very light weight in the beginning and work yourself up to where your legs are strong and you will see a huge difference.

Chapter 8

HERBAL TREATMENTS & SUPPLEMENTS

Below are the facts and the supplements that I researched and found to have been instrumental in curing my cancer. I will explain each fact and supplement and why they work and also give you some websites to go to for more in-depth information for those of you who require more information and proof. When you read this you will see that it all makes perfect sense. This is what worked for me. I see no reason why it shouldn't work for you. The following are everything that I took to eliminate my prostate cancer. The short list is IP6 with Inositol, Flor-Essence (Essiac) Tea, Budwig Diet, OncoPLEX, CELLFOOD, maitake mushroom, ALAmar, Avemar, CELLFOOD DNA-RNA Cell Regeneration Formula, Lycopene, pomegranate extract, Vitamins E and C, Resveratrol, fruits and nuts. I would say the first five for sure but the rest are for added and expedient results. And in case the thought crossed your mind, I, in no way, get paid for making these recommendations or was ever asked by anyone to make these recommendations. These are just the things that I discovered on my own that worked for me and I am passing them along to you.

CELLFOOD - Cancer and Oxygen

Cancer cells cannot survive in the presence of high levels of oxygen. *Healthy cells* cannot survive in an oxygen *deprived* state. (http://www.healingdaily.com/conditions/cancer-and-oxygen.htm) It's kind of like your lawn. If you don't water your lawn the healthy grass dies and weeds take its place. So you must get your body and your cells oxygenated. There is a product out on the market called CELLFOOD. What it does is use the water in your body to make oxygen within your body since water is made up of one part hydrogen and two parts oxygen. The chemical compound in CELLFOOD reacts with a minute amount water in your body and splits the oxygen atom from the hydrogen atom (of $H2O$) to make the oxygen for your cells. Also, there is a health benefit for the hydrogen atom too as it reacts like hydrogen peroxide within your body. All this is detailed out in the CELLFOOD website: www.cellfood.com. Another huge benefit that CELLFOOD has is it makes your body more pH balanced. In their website they attribute eliminating lactic acids to athletic performance and muscle rebuilding. In our instance, CELLFOOD is helping to eliminate the lactic acids that cancer cells cause when fermenting sugar. As we now know, the fermented sugar makes your body more acidic as I detailed out in the last chapter.

To understand why some tissues in the body are deficient in oxygen and therefore prone to cancer, it is helpful to understand the nature of acidity and alkalinity in the body too. As mentioned in Chapter 6, cancerous tissues are acidic, whereas healthy tissues are alkaline. It is important to keep your body in an alkaline state to prevent and to cure cancer. Here is a website for all the foods we eat and what they do as far as helping our bodies to be either acidic or alkaline: http://acidalkalinediet.com/listofalkalinefoods.pdf. Also, you can take a tablespoon of Apple Cider Vinegar every day to keep your body in an alkaline state. Potassium

Bicarbonate with water is good too for helping to create alkalinity in your body.

For a little more on the technical side of why oxygenating your body and putting it into an alkaline state works please read the following: This is from the website that I gave you in Chapter 6: www.healingdaily. com/conditions/saliva-ph-test.htm. Water decomposes into H+ and OH-. When a solution contains more H+ than OH- then it is said to be acidic. When it contains more OH- than H+ then it is said to be alkaline. This is because the negative ion in the OH attracts a positive electrical charge from minerals in your body which creates an alkalinity state in your body and the reverse is true with the positively charged H ion. Also, when oxygen enters an acid solution it can combine with H+ ions to form water. The oxygen helps to neutralize the acid, while at the same time the acid prevents oxygen from reaching the tissues that need it. Acidic tissues are devoid of free oxygen. An alkaline solution is just the reverse. Two hydroxyl ions (OH-) can combine to produce one water molecule and one oxygen atom. In other words, an alkaline solution can provide oxygen to the tissues.

The pH scale goes from 0 to 14, with 7 being neutral. Below 7 is acidic and above 7 is alkaline. The blood, lymph nodes and cerebral spinal fluid in the human body are designed to be slightly alkaline at a pH of 7.4. Body pH is a very important topic as you can see. More about the role of oxygen in fighting cancer can be found here http://www.healingdaily.com/conditions/cancer-and-oxygen.htm.

Special Note: In this hyperlink it talks about drinking food grade hydrogen peroxide. I have recently started using this protocol although I didn't use hydrogen peroxide while I was curing myself. It was only after I was cured that I experimented with it simply for preventive maintenance as well as internal and cellular cleansing. Had I known about it before I would have used it in my protocol because claims are that using hydrogen peroxide will clean out the dead cancer cells from your body along with oxygenating your body. But as of this writing I do not know enough about it to make any further claims or testaments so use it at your own risk if you want. For more information you can go to this site: www.foodgrade-hydrogenperoxide.com.

I also introduced another CELLFOOD Product into my regime called CELLFOOD DNA-RNA. This is a cell *regenerating* product. I felt that as I was killing off cancer cells that I needed to enhance the health of my good cells to take over where the cancer cells were. So I added this to my routine about a year into my program. I don't know if it did any good but I felt better knowing that I was doing as much as I could to regenerate my good cells. Plus, from what I read about CELLFOOD DNA-RNA, it is a good anti-aging product to restore our DNA methyl groups which we start losing at the age of around 25. I want to keep as much as I can no matter what it is if I had it when I was younger. I think that is one of the secrets to longevity.

Budwig Recipe

The Budwig Recipe is probably one of the most important staples of my program if not THE most important. I started eating this Budwig Recipe early on in my cancer fight. I feel that I obtained remarkable results from it. I stumbled upon it by accident. It was while I was doing searches on the internet looking for natural cancer cures. As you may or may not know, within a lot of internet searches there are hyperlinks to other sites that relate to what you happen to be reading. They're usually just explanations or definitions of specific words that you are reading at the time. However, during one of these searches up pops this website on the Budwig Diet from one of the hyperlinks that I clicked on. I was floored when I read it because I never ever heard of this Budwig Diet or Budwig Protocol. But there it was and I called my wife in to read it with me. We were very excited having stumbled on this and also very mystified. Was this an act of G-d having brought me to this site? It sure seemed like it.

I don't want to get too technical with you and bore you to death or cause you to skip ahead so I am only going to just give you the gist on the theory of this Budwig Recipe. I get lost and bored myself when I start reading the technical stuff so I don't want to do that to you here. I will provide you with the links at the end of this segment to find the technical jargon in case you do want to delve even further into the technical aspects as to why it works.

Dr. Johanna Budwig, a German biochemist, found that the blood of seriously ill cancer patients was deficient in certain important essential ingredients which included substances called phosphatides and lipoproteins, while the blood of a healthy person always contains sufficient quantities of these essential ingredients of the blood. She found that when these natural ingredients were reintroduced into the body over approximately a three month period, tumors gradually receded, weakness and anemia disappeared and life energy was restored. Symptoms of cancer, liver dysfunction and diabetes were alleviated. I have been eating it going on 2 years now. However, I am at a maintenance level right now, eating it only about 3-4 times a week, once a day. I actually like the fact that I can eat this for breakfast in place of a regular breakfast meal. It is filling, nutritious and replenishes the ingredients that are needed in our bodies to kill and ward off cancer. What more can you ask for? Also, the alternative is usually bad for you like sugary cereals, waffles and pancakes, as well as pork products in breakfast meals that are fatty and carcinogenic.

Dr. Budwig applied this discovery in clinical trials by feeding cancer patients a mixture of 3-6 tbsps. of flaxseed oil and 4 oz. (1/2 cup) low-fat cottage cheese daily. The mixture is created by mixing the flaxseed oil and low-fat cottage cheese thoroughly, blending it together into a *water-soluble* mixture. This is important since water and oil don't normally mix together. But when this sulphurated protein in the cottage cheese is blended together with the flaxseed oil a chemical reaction happens and this mixture now becomes water soluble and easier to digest and gets into your system faster and easier. You can add pineapple, blueberries or other fruit to improve the taste but I used concentrated pomegranate extract since it claims to be a great cancer fighter as well.

There are a number of different measurements that are suggested in various websites that I reviewed for this recipe. However, I settled on using 3 tablespoons of *cold pressed* flaxseed oil (I used Barlean's in the refrigerator section of a health food store) 6 tablespoons of organic cottage cheese, one tablespoon of organic yogurt (the yogurt and the additional liquid "whey" that comes together in the organic yogurt help to make the mixture smoother and not so thick) and about 1 to 2 tablespoons of pomegranate extract syrup. Some websites suggested using honey. I did this at first and it made the Budwig Recipe tolerable and not too bad tasting actually. However, the Budwig Recipe does require an acquired taste. Please don't let this deter you. You will acquire the taste and it will be fine. But then I read up on honey. Honey is still a form of sugar and I would suggest that you refrain from using any sweeteners in this protocol that I am laying out for you. As I mentioned earlier, sugar feeds cancer cells so I wanted nothing to keep those cancer cells alive within me. So instead of using honey I switched to Pomegranate Extract.

I use a regular "wand type" mixer that has a mushroom shaped head at the end of it for easier mixing and blending. You can get a mixing kit that has the blender and a compatible mixing container together. I blend the mixture together (except the pomegranate extract) until it looks creamy like a mayonnaise texture. It usually takes 2 to 3 minutes of blending to get it to this texture. Then I add the pomegranate extract and blend it all together for about another minute.

Now you are ready to grind the flax seeds. I did this in a small coffee bean grinder. I measured 2 tablespoons of whole flax seeds and poured them into the grinder. You don't want to use flax seeds that are pre-ground and you don't want to grind up a whole bunch at one time as they say flax seeds get "rancid" after a few hours of grinding them up. I ground them up for 1 to 2 minutes until they were all ground up into a powdery mixture. Then I poured these ground flax seeds in with the mixture of flaxseed oil, cottage cheese and Pomegranate Extract. I mixed it up with a long stemmed spoon and now it was ready to eat. I ate this twice a day for the first four months, at which point I got my second biopsy. That is when I got the first good news in all this. I continued to eat it twice a day but there were some days that I missed and only ate it once a day for the following 6 months. I continued this until my fifth biopsy in May of 2010. That's when there was no cancer to be found after the 24 core biopsy. From there I went to the maintenance plan.

In the website, it also suggests that "seriously ill" patients should drink a glass of champagne when eating the flaxseed oil and cottage cheese mixture. I decided that whether I was seriously ill or not I was going to give it everything that I could to fight this cancer. I found a really nice, inexpensive brand of champagne called Charles De Fere, from France. I only paid about ten dollars a bottle and it was surprisingly good! Not your cheap fruity tasting brand or bitter tasting kind either. I bought this until I could not find it anymore. I then came across a good deal on a case of Veuve Clicquot Ponsardin. So, every night for about 3 months I drank a glass of this champagne (along with my wife ☺) and it was just one of the more pleasurable perks of this program. Quite a nice perk I might add. I would highly recommend that when first starting out on this program that you go out and buy some nice champagne to drink with the Budwig recipe. There is a medical and scientific reason to drink it. Please read up more on this in the web links below. For more technical information on the

Budwig Recipe please go to: http://www.cancure.org/budwig_diet.htm (there is an underscore between "budwig" and "diet") and http://www.mnwelldir.org/docs/cancer1/budwig.htm. Plus I would also encourage you to do a search on your own for Budwig Diet and Budwig Recipe. You can even find some other sites by searching Budwig *Protocol*, too. Here, also, is a great video for you to watch as well... http://www.youtube.com/watch?v= RSoddptWL0s

Essiac Tea

Essiac tea, I feel, is the number two most important supplement in my regimen. Essiac tea is a combination of herbs and roots that was developed by the Ojibwa Indians in Canada many years ago. The Ojibwa Indians might sound familiar because of Shania Twain's involvement with the Ojibwa Indians in Canada. A nurse named Rene Caisse brought it to the attention of the Canadian medical community back in the 1930's and '40's when she learned about it from a prospector's wife who had breast cancer and was cured from this assortment of Herbs and Roots. This assortment of roots and herbs consisted of Burdock Root, Slippery Elm, Inner Bark, Sheep Sorrel and Indian Rhubarb Root.

I first found out about Essiac tea when I read about Flor-Essence Tea in the *Natural Cancer Cures* book. When I showed this to my wife she said that is what she drank when she had a bad Pap test that showed Pre-Cancerous cells in her uterus. She drank this tea and the precancerous cells went away. When she told me that that is when I knew that I had to incorporate this into my regimen.

Flor-Essence has all the ingredients that Essiac tea has except that they added a few more herbs. They added Watercress, Blessed Thistle, Red Clover and Kelp. Since I read that these herbs individually helped in treating cancer I felt like they probably would help in the Essiac formula as well.

At first, I drank 3 ounces mixed in 6 ounces of hot *purified* water twice a day for the first 6 months. Then I cut back to 2 ounces with 6 ounces of purified water. In the beginning I bought the pre-made liquid but that got to be pretty expensive. So I decided that I was going to make my own because Flor-Essence comes in boxes of pre-measured packs of the raw crushed herbs. I thought that this was better, too, because there was residue left over in the mixture after I made it. I felt like this was a better and more powerful concentrate than what I could buy. Plus, it was cheaper. I had saved the bottles from the pre-made liquids that I had bought in the beginning because they are brown tinted bottles that keep the boiled mixture that I made fresher and from breaking down too quickly. They are just the right measurements that the boiled mixtures need as well.

IP6 with Inositol

I heard about IP6 with Inositol in the *Natural Cancer Cures* book. IP6 with Inositol is supposed to boost your immune system as well as the Natural Killer Cells within your body. I never heard of Natural Killer Cells before. Actually, there were a lot of things that I hadn't heard of before I put myself on this venture. This is just one more. But it just made common sense to me that your immune system needs to be at its peak to be able to fight these cancer cells. So I took this IP6 w/ Inositol to do just that. For just a little technical background on this, I will give you just enough information in hopes that it will back up my reasoning to use it. Natural Killer Cells are cells that can react against and destroy another cell without prior sensitization to it. Natural Killer (NK) Cells are part of our first line of defense against cancer cells and virus-infected cells. NK cells are small lymphocytes that originate in the bone marrow and develop fully in the absence of the thymus (which atrophies as you grow into adulthood). NK cells look for a "banner" flown by normal cells. If the NK cell recognizes the "banner," it spares that cell. If the "banner" is absent, the NK cell attaches to the target cell, releases a burst of chemicals that penetrate the target cell's wall and the target cell breaks up (lyzes). This is as technical as I will get on this subject. You can go on Wikipedia and spend about 2 days just trying to look up and understand just exactly what the science is behind Natural Killer Cells but I don't think that is really necessary. Just know that IP6 w/ Inositol helps boost the killer cells that attack cancer cells and kills them.

I got the powder form as that is supposed to be 6 times more powerful than the tablets or capsules. I would drink a glass in the morning right when I woke up and one right when I went to bed. This is because it says that IP6 with Inositol is best taken on an empty stomach. And don't get fooled into buying just IP6 without the inositol just because it is cheaper. The inositol is what activates that drug. I would buy Cell Forte' as that seems to be the best according to my research.

I also heard in an NBC Today show segment that inositol alone was good for defeating lung cancer in particular. I was very excited when I heard about this discovery. That meant to me that I was doing the right thing and I was way ahead of the game. For more on the technical information on this supplement you can go to http://jn.nutrition.org/ content/133/11/3778S.full on the web.

Maitake Mushroom

Another supplement that I read about in *Natural Cancer Cures,* that I took, was Maitake Mushroom. There are a few different versions of this herbal supplement. The one that I went with was of course the most expensive... Grifron-Pro Maitake D Fraction 4x. I read up on this and I researched it and to me it made a lot of sense to take it. Keep in mind that I was on a short time schedule. I had four months before I was to go back to Mayo and have the prostatectomy. So I was throwing the kitchen sink at this cancer to see what kind of results I could get in this relatively short period of time. Since prostate cancer is a slow growing cancer, in my mind, if it took a long time to get to the point that it was at then it was going to take a long time to cure too. So I wanted all the supplements that I could find to cure myself and the most powerful too. Maitake D Fraction 4x was the most powerful so I bought that. I would just caution you to be careful when buying this supplement because it is easy to get it mixed up with the other strengths on the market and you can easily end up with the low dosage at a much cheaper cost and that is where you may get tripped up. You think that you are getting a good deal on this supplement when in reality you are getting a low strength version. I took 2 to

3 tablets in the morning and 2 to 3 tablets in the evening, along with all the other supplements that I took at this time. I took this religiously for the first 4 months and then *consistently* (maybe missed here and there) for about the next 4 months after that; when by that time I had already gone through 4 biopsies. At that 8 month point I dropped the maitake mushroom. It was about $100 a bottle so I tried leaving it out of my regime from that point and I seemed to do OK without it as I am cancer free now. So I would leave it up to you. If you think that you might want to try everything else first, try going without it between biopsies and see what results you get since this is probably the most expensive supplement of them all. If it was me, I would still use it as I would want to do everything possible, at least in the beginning, to cure myself and get myself started on the right path.

There is another mushroom extract that I have recently found out about that is supposed to be more powerful that maitake mushroom and that is ABM Mushroom from Brazil. I never used it myself, however. I just found this while on the International Wellness Directory (www. mnwelldir.org) website that I gave you at the end of the Budwig Recipe section under the *hydrazine sulphate* hyperlink. This goes to show you what else you can find while researching.

Lycopene

This is a derivative of tomatoes. I hated tomatoes and never ate them except for pizza and spaghetti. Maybe that is one of the reasons for the prostate cancer. Who knows! But with Lycopene, I can give my prostate the nutrient that it may have needed the most. Lycopene is supposed to be better for the prostate than even Saw Palmetto. So I took this as part of the pill supplements that I took twice a day. Ironically, I never took Saw Palmetto in this treatment which is probably THE most common supplement on the market that people take for the health of their prostate. I had taken it on a regular basis though before I knew that I had prostate cancer. I guess that is why I didn't take it while I was trying to treat myself. I had lost faith in it. Lately, I have come across some good subsequent information on Saw Palmetto, though. So it is up to you whether you want to add it to your regimen. Now this is for prostate cancer. You may have a different cancer so you may or may not decide this is right for you in your specific case.

OncoPLEX

OncoPLEX was introduced to me by my anti-aging doctor, Dr. Douglas Hall. OncoPLEX is a derivative of broccoli sprouts and/or broccoli seeds. I ate a lot of fresh broccoli, mostly with the fresh salads that I ate when I was heavy into my cancer treatment.

The technical term for this supplement is Sulforaphane glucosinolate. It is the precursor to the chemical, sulforaphane, which is produced in your body when you eat cruciferous vegetables like broccoli. Sulforaphane triggers the production of enzymes that help detoxify cancer causing chemicals. So OncoPLEX is another herbal supplement in the use of detoxification and also enhances the antioxidant process in your body to fight free radical damage.

ALAmax CR

ALAmax CR is a form of ALA or Alpha Lipoic Acid. It is a powerful, whole-body, multi-functional antioxidant that helps create and maintain healthy well-functioning cells. ALAmax CR is designed to neutralize free radicals at the moment of their formation - before they can cause damage to your cells. ALAmax CR has the ability to destroy free radicals in both water-based and lipid-based cells, making it the ideal whole-body antioxidant. In addition, ALAmax CR increases the levels of the body's own master detoxifier (glutathione) by a full 30%. ALAmax CR also "regenerates" other consumable antioxidants, such as vitamin C, E, and CoQ10, giving them the ability to continue fighting free radicals for extended periods of time.

Alpha Lipoic Acid is found naturally in every cell in the body. So my thinking was, if ALA is found naturally in all my cells then I am going to add more to what is naturally already there. I may have been suffering from low quantities which caused my cells to weaken and fall susceptible to cancer. In any case, I was going to add ALA to my regimen. It couldn't hurt. Besides, ALA is touted to help reduce fat in body tissue. So if nothing else, I was going lose body fat. Coupled with that, ALA is an anti-oxidant as well. This coincides with my attempts at longevity and eliminating free radicals. So that was another plus for this supplement.

AVEMAR

Avemar is a B vitamin derivative of wheat germ. It helps promote a healthy immune system as well as being a cancer fighter. The website for this supplement is careful in its wording as far as being a cancer fighter. It is apparent that the clinical trials are still going on and they don't want to claim that it is specifically a cancer fighting supplement.

My functional doctor turned me onto this supplement so I tried it in about the sixth month of my self-treatment (even though what I had been doing was working quite well). I did 60 days of this as it comes in boxes of 30 packets for a one month treatment. The only problem that I was facing was the need to take this on an empty stomach and not eat for 3 hours. It seems that everything was telling me to take on an empty stomach and there are only so many opportunities to have an empty stomach. So with all the other supplements needing to be taken on an empty stomach and then not eating for 3 hours what I had to do was get up at 2 am and take this. That was not always easy to do so; that's why I only did it for 60 days. But again, I was willing to try everything so I included this into my program on a limited basis.

Other Supplements

I took a whole host of other vitamins and supplements and most of them I was taking before I even knew that I had cancer. I was taking Resveratrol, Cold pressed Fish Oil for Omega 3's, Co-Q-10, Vitamins E and C, Selenium, and Glucosamine with Chondroitin. These were designed to help me with my anti-aging program. I still take them to assist with the anti-aging process.

Chapter 9

MORE ON MY EXPERIENCE

After I had the 24 core biopsy in June of the first year that I was on this regimen, I will be the first to admit that I slacked off a bit on my own protocol. Instead of taking my supplements, Budwig and Essiac Tea religiously and instead of maintaining a strict diet, I faltered. The results were so great in such a short amount of time I figured that all I had to do was coast to the finish line. WRONG!

I waited for 6 months and instead of going back to Dr. Taub, I decided that this time I was going back to Mayo. But I was going back there with arrogance. I was going to go back there to prove them wrong; to prove to them that I didn't have to have the surgery like they suggested. I had cured my cancer so *in your face*. I scheduled an Executive Physical like I do every year and was going to get everything done all at once. So on November 11th I went to Mayo. The first thing that I did when I got to Mayo, like I always do, is get my blood drawn. You have to fast from the night before and nothing but water in the morning to obscure the test results. I always get my testosterone tested too just for the record. I was off all the testosterone and I wanted to see what my physician thought of where my results were. I always go to see my attending physician there at Mayo before my biopsies just to see how everything is. When I saw Dr. Rodriguez he went over all my preliminary test results and the only thing that I was interested in was my PSA at this point. And it was really good news. It was now down to 1.28. Wow, this is the lowest that it had been in two years. I was really happy and excited. Dr. Rodriguez just fluffed it off though. It was still over a 1.0 so in his estimation I still had the same amount of cancer that I always had. In my mind I thought he was crazy. There is no way that I could have it as bad as it showed the last time that I took tests here. I was very optimistic.

So, as I was preparing for my fourth biopsy of the year I asked the biopsy technician if he had ever heard of anyone curing prostate cancer. He told me that he had been working at Mayo for 12 years and had never heard of anyone curing prostate cancer before. I told him, "Well, you are about to see it now" and I gave him a very confident smile. Because, of course, if my results in June showed only two of the twenty four cores having cancer cells and my PSA test was 1.4 then I had to have completely cured it by now. I have heard of other guys with PSA test in the teens and didn't have prostate cancer so I thought that since my PSA was continuing to fall (to a 1.28) and my results were so good when I did my last biopsy with the 1.4 PSA that there was no way that they were going to find any cancer left in me this time.

Of course, I was wrong. According to the Mayo examine three of the ten cores showed cancer cells and one of them showed 60% of the sample containing cancer cells. "What the…???" I was pretty stunned to say the least. I couldn't believe it and of course I was recommended to still have the surgery. As bad as I initially felt that these tests were, I was inclined to agree with them. It had been almost a year that I had been on my routine and the cancer seemed to have come back from where it was in June. This was ridiculous. Then I started thinking to myself, "Wait a minute, this is still good news. I don't have nearly the amount of cancer that they found last time, my Gleason Scores were now all consistent 6's instead of some 7's AND my PSA scores have continued to fall every time that I took a blood test. All this added up to what I was doing WAS working. Of course the results weren't nearly as good as I would have expected but never the less they were better than a year ago and that is what counts. So I decided it was time to quit being a slacker and get back on the strict regimen that I was on at the beginning of the year. Then I would have a blood test in February to see where I was in the scheme of things and then another biopsy in March.

Well, I couldn't wait until February, three months after this last test. I had an idea. I called Dr. Hall and made an appointment to see him. I asked him to write out a prescription for a PSA test and a testosterone level test and I asked him to put me back on testosterone. I was really dragging butt now as it had been a year since I had been off my testosterone replacement therapy. I wanted to find out where I was with my testosterone levels and also get back on it so I felt better. When I meet with Dr. Hall again after all this time being off testosterone, he had a *new lease on thought,* as he had reconsidered what he subscribed to as the traditional way of thinking. That was, that testosterone was fuel to cancer. To put it in his original terms, "It was like throwing gasoline on the fire". Now he was thinking more in the direction that I had always thought, and that was, twenty and thirty something men just don't get prostate cancer and they have a huge amount of testosterone flowing in their veins. So there must be something to the effect of testosterone *preventing* cancer, not fueling it.

Well, good news, bad news. The bad news was that my testosterone levels were in the toilet just like I thought. Now I know that this is very controversial and I cannot legally advocate that everyone do this, but I thought, why not experiment on myself. The good news was that my PSA was now down to 1.1. That was such good news I could have cried. I practically skipped out of Dr. Hall's office when he gave me the news. It seemed that with me getting back onto a strict schedule of my own prescribed routine, it was doing a lot of good. But now I was going to take it one step further and that was experiment for a month and take the testosterone consistently and see what if anything that the testosterone does to my PSA levels as I was scheduled to do another blood test with Dr Taub in February anyway. In this next chapter I will go into testosterone replacement therapy a little more in depth.

Chapter 10

HORMONE REPLACEMENT THERAPY

When I found out that I had prostate cancer I was incredibly mad at Dr. Hall, my Functional (Anti-Aging) Doctor. I thought, "He had to have known that this was going to *cause* cancer". All of this was his fault. I got off testosterone immediately. After consulting with Dr. Hall he even agreed that it was like "pouring gasoline on the fire". But, after 9 months of being off testosterone I was back to being tired, irritable and not thinking clearly at all. I was a miserable person. I talked to my wife about it. I told her that I thought that I needed to get back on testosterone. I talked again to Dr. Hall about it as well. To my surprise he had a changed opinion of testosterone for a cancer patient. He told me about a book called *"Testosterone For Life"* by Dr. Abraham Morgentaler. Dr. Morgentaler is a professor at Harvard University and a practicing urologist in Boston. Dr. Morgentaler disputes that using bio-identical testosterone is a death sentence for cancer patients. He goes on to explain that the evidence and the research are flawed and he explains why it is flawed. Even today there are articles coming out in the newspaper saying that the common practice of chemical castration (such as Lupron injections) for prostate cancer patients is being rethought and discontinued by a lot of doctors. There are even television ads now that are promoting testosterone replacement for "Low T" which you never would have heard a year ago. But with that said, my brother didn't like the thought of me getting back on testosterone and neither did any of my other doctors. But I, my wife, and my Functional Doctor all thought that it was a good idea for me to go back on testosterone and we would just keep a close eye on my PSA levels and see what affect it had on my biopsies. So, for the sake of my quality of life as well as proving the other doctors wrong (yet again) after 6 months I am happy to say that I was still feeling great and my PSA had steadily *dropped*. It went from a 1.28 in November, around the time that I started back on testosterone replacement, to a 1.0 in April. So as I am still on the road to recovery I feel that the testosterone is partly to thank for the recovery that I am experiencing.

I thought about this from a common sense point of view and I ask you to think about this too. Young men whose testosterone levels are at their highest in their 20's and 30's rarely develop prostate cancer or any other cancers for that matter like you do when you get older. I think that when you start *losing* your hormones, both men and women, it triggers something in your body that says you are no longer a (re)productive member of society and you are no longer needed on this earth. So your body starts to shut down and you come down with all sorts of ailments due to low hormone levels, including cancer. I know that this goes against all of today's wisdom from the medical gurus out there but I am just telling you what has worked for me and worked very well for me.

If you were to read *The Calcium Factor* 2 and *The One Minute Cure* 9 you will find that they both explain what I thought all along, that the pharmaceutical companies have a conspiracy going to keep news like what is in this book out of the public domain. Basically, if it can't be patented then the pharmaceutical companies cannot protect their interests and then there is no money to be made. I would recommend reading these books that, I feel, back up what my hypothesis is. I feel the same way about a lot of doctors too... that they are just in it for the money, not for the patient's best interest. And I say "a lot" but not all. Some doctors are coming around to this way of thinking and are embracing it and studying it and those are the doctors that will be in business 20 years from now. There is a good article on this in Reader's Digest (October 2011).

Doctors need to change with the times. But, those doctors that are resistant to change, that are of the mindset that if they can't make any money off a protocol or if there is even a risk of them not being able to make any money, they are going to reject any theory that goes against their medical *"business"*. And curing oneself naturally and staying healthy does not necessarily help a doctor's medical practice. It hurts their *business*. And that seems to be the bottom line with a lot of doctors in my opinion. But again, not all and not the ones that stuck with me like Dr. Hall and Dr. Taub. But I cannot think of any other reason why a lot of them reject this method of cure other than the money aspect. A family member of mines' doctors is a perfect example. They would not approve the Essiac tea and Budwig Protocol even though these are just natural food grade supplements and herbs. Ignorance is a terrible thing. Her doctors, unlike my doctors, were not going to approve this since they knew nothing about it. So, seek second and third opinions when you are dealing with your life. Don't take no for an answer... like I didn't.

Chapter 11

<u>FALLEN PEOPLE</u>

As I am writing this book, I am witnessing many celebrities passing away. Some like Farrah Fawcett, Patrick Swazye, Dennis Hopper, Elizabeth Edwards and I think that the one that affected me the most was Steve Jobs since he was into holistic cures. He just never found the right protocol like I did. I just wanted to reach out to them and say "Hey, I've got the answer, listen to me". I even tried to contact Farrah Fawcett to tell her about my cancer treatment program. I wrote People Magazine and the Today Show and no one ever got back with me. I guess they thought that I was a quack or some nut who just wanted contact with a celebrity. It was just so sad not knowing how to reach out to these folks. That is a big reason why I decided to write this book; to relay this information in book form and to give myself some sort of credibility with people.

I take this program to heart and if you need some further information or if you need some further assistance with this plan, I will be happy to talk to you to help you get set up on this plan because I don't want people to give up. I want people to get cured and cured completely. I do not want people to die anymore like so many have already. This is the way to go, not chemotherapy and radiation. Chemotherapy and radiation may (or may not) kill the cancer but it may kill you in the process as well. Not only that but, it is only a temporary cure. If you don't get to the core of the issue then the cancer will be back. I am even concerned about Michael Douglas. As of this writing he has said that he is cured of cancer but I fear that it will be back if he hasn't done the steps that I have outlined in this book. He needs to put his body in the state that it needs to be in to withstand any possibility of the cancer returning.

I have reached out to a lot of personal friends, friends of friends and even family members and a lot of them have a hard time accepting this advice. They depended on doctors to tell them what the best source of treatment is and most doctors only use the conventional way that they were taught in medical school and, as I mentioned, is best for their medical practice. Maybe a good many of you are asking yourselves, "Why does Ira Miller think that he is smarter than a doctor?" It's not that I think that I am smarter than a doctor. It's like I told you in the last chapter, a good many doctors are in medicine to make money. It is their business. (Don't forget to read "The One Minute Cure" and "The Calcium Factor") I have taken the common sense approach to all this and researched what the Good L-rd put in my head to research and came up with what worked to cure my cancer. So it's faith, research and common sense that got me cured and got this book written.

Not to keep beating a dead horse but this is the way that I look at it: As I said in the beginning of this book and then again in the last chapter; doctors, hospitals, Big Pharma(ceuticals), medical appliance companies, medical machinery companies, and even the offshoots like the insurance industry and the cancer institutes, would be drastically affected if we all kept ourselves healthy through common sense practices like diet, exercise, cleansing and hormone replacement therapy or cured ourselves naturally. Think about it; many of them would be out of business or at least trimmed down to a much smaller level. It is a known fact that Big Pharma employs thousands of pharmaceutical reps to woo the doctors to use their products. Big Pharma is one of the biggest lobbyists in the nation too. They make billions and billions of dollars every year on their products that would not be needed if we only changed our lifestyles and didn't abuse our bodies. So you are not going to hear about this way of curing yourself through the traditional channels of the medical community. It is against the very nature that supports their way of life.

You may ask yourself, "How come I have not heard about any of this until now?" Well, the answer is, natural supplements and herbs, a good diet and cleansing cannot be patented and made money on. So you will never hear these things advertised like you do with all of these pharmaceutical drugs. Doctors are not going to promote it either because they get a residual from the prescriptions that they write. Have you ever wondered why it is that when you go to the doctor and he or she prescribes an antibiotic it is not the same one that you had last time? It is because you are given what the pharmaceuticals are asking the doctors to prescribe at the time. This is why you have not heard about this curative treatment up until now. There is no money to be made like there is in pharmaceutical drugs and medical treatments. And that is why a lot of your cancer research organizations do not tout this method of treatment. Most of them are backed by the big pharmaceutical companies and they are in *business* (even as a non-profit) to find a pharmaceutical cure not a natural cure. They want to find that magic pill you can take and be cured when in reality this natural cure is the best cure where you will stay cured. That is what is wrong with America today. Americans just want a quick fix. So these are the incentives not to embrace this cure.

Chapter 12

<u>RADIATION & CHEMOTHERAPY</u>

As I have mentioned, I cured my cancer with no surgery, radiation, chemotherapy treatments or pharmaceutical drugs. The main problem with radiation and chemotherapy is that there is a lot of collateral damage or "side effects" as they are liked to be called. To me it is like setting a bomb off in your body to kill your target but along with that target there are a lot of other things damaged within the field of range in that area. Some of that can be devastating to those collateral areas. You can get all or a few of these "side effects" but they all are counterproductive as far as I am concerned. However, I cannot believe the amount of people that I have come across that elect to go this route only because a doctor has told them that there is no other way. This is unfortunate and I welcome the day when we look back and see how radiation and chemotherapy was so extremely barbaric. It may be 50 years and it may be 100 years from now but we will look back in history one day and realize how barbaric these techniques are just like we look back today, 50 or 100 years and see how antiquated those techniques were back then.

With radiation, since it cannot be targeted to only the cancer tumor or cancer cells, there is that area around the tumor and cancer cells that is affected. In the case of prostate cancer, when you radiate the prostate you burn the whole prostate along with the nerve bundles that run along the outside of the prostate that serve for erections as well as the bladder that is touching the prostate. So as my own doctors explained to me, if I had radiation treatment I could never have my prostate removed in the future without having to have a colostomy bag for the rest of my life. I would have to have a portion of my bladder removed along with the prostate and possibly never have an erection again either. This is because the prostate would have been so badly burned that it would literally be burnt and scarred to the bladder wall. Needless to say, this could lead to problems with urination as well as, as I mentioned, erections. It was also revealed to me by my doctors that there may not be an immediate effect on erections but down the road, years later, those nerves would eventually succumb to the radiation effects. So for all this, I decided that radiation was not for me.

I also know someone who had radiation for esophageal cancer. A world renowned cancer hospital administered the radiation on the tumor in their throat. Well, this person, literally, could not eat for some time after that. Not only that but months later, after the tumor was gone in their throat, they had problems swallowing because of all the scar tissue that had resulted from the burning of the throat and esophagus. They then had to go back into the hospital and have a stretching tool stuck down the inside of their throat so the throat could be stretched so food would not lodge in the throat anymore. And even after going through all this the cancer returned and they gave this person six months to live and told them that there was nothing more that could be done. Fortunately, they did not listen to this cancer hospital and they went elsewhere and were treated with more conventional options like chemotherapy and radiation again. Again the cancer went away only to return once more with it being in their lymph nodes now. I am hoping at this point that this person will listen to reason and decide that the program that I have described in this book is the only way to become completely healthy again. But this is a perfect example as to why you want to heal your body naturally and put it in the state that it needs to be in to kill the cancer that is in your body and not allow the cancer to turn up somewhere else. Plus, the collateral damage can be devastating.

As far as chemotherapy goes, it is designed to target the fast growing cancer cells in your body but it also targets other cells in your body too. This is like dropping a "nuclear" bomb off in your body as it pretty much destroys your entire immune system and causes other damaging effects as well. B*oosting* your immune system, not killing it, is pretty much what my program that I have laid out here is predicated on. A strong immune system wards off any future cancer once you have removed the cancer from your body and eradicated the source of that cancer. Simply by eliminating sugar from your diet, oxygenating your cells and putting your cells into an alkaline state does pretty much what chemotherapy does but without the side effects.

Chemotherapy can cause problems like Neutropenia, which is low white blood cell count. Low white blood cell count will leave you prone to infections. That alone can kill someone. Have you ever heard of someone going to the hospital for minor surgery only to end up dying due to an infection that they contracted in the hospital? Then there is Anemia, which is low red blood cell count. Low red blood cell count is bad because your red blood cells are what carry oxygen throughout your body. As I have mentioned, cancer cannot survive in an oxygenated body. If your red blood cells are compromised then you are not helping your body kill cancer cells the way that it was really designed to. Next, there is Thrombocytopenia, which is low platelet count. Low platelet blood counts can result in bruising or internal bleeding. These are some of the more severe problems that you may have from chemotherapy. Some of the less severe, but equally as inconvenient, is hair loss, loss of energy, mouth sores, pain, diarrhea and/or constipation. So personally, I would not have radiation and/or chemotherapy but even if you did decide to have radiation and/or chemotherapy you should complement that with this holistic treatment to get your body back to a healthy condition as soon as possible. And that includes cleansing as soon as possible to get those poisons from the radiation and chemotherapy out of your body. You will bounce back a lot sooner and you will raise your resistance to a reoccurrence of your cancer or other cancers within your body.

Chapter 13

<u>IN CONCLUSION</u>

Not only has this program that I put myself on cured my prostate cancer but it has made my whole body healthy. Today, through my change in lifestyle and leading a healthy life I feel that I am healthier now than I have ever been in my entire adult life. I look in the mirror and I do not see the wrinkles on my face that I saw there 2 years ago. I have people tell me that I look great all the time. I have people tell me that I look like I am in my early 40's. The dark age spots that I saw on my hands two years ago are no longer there. I have not had a bout with skin cancer since I started this program of curing my prostate cancer. When I started this program I was wearing a size 33 pants and they were getting really tight. Today my size 32 pants are getting loose on me. So now that I have cured my cancer I am not going to go back to my old eating lifestyle of eating red meat 4 nights a week and eating sweets and chocolate every night although sweets are probably the hardest thing to stay away from, especially at night. I know now that sugar is a killer and I will continue to do my best to stay away from it for the rest of my life. But will I abstain from it 100%? I can honestly say no… as long as I am cancer free. On limited occasions I will treat myself. But if for some reason the cancer were to come back I would absolutely discontinue all ingestion of sweets and sugars. I will continue to stay away from red meat though as it has all those additives that I feel can trigger cancer in me. There could be the occasional rib-eye steak though… I have to be honest. But again, this is as long as I continue not to have cancer.

The bottom line is, to be cancer free we need to do and have a few things going on. We need to have our bodies in sync. Our bodies need to be oxygenated, free from pesticides (cleansing) and sugar and pH balanced. Also, our immunity system needs to be at optimum level. We need to exercise on a continuing basis and we need to have the proper diet. By doing all this, that is what is going to keep me cancer free. By following this program I should never have to worry about having or getting cancer ever again. On top of that, I am confident that I should have very few ailments that I would normally have had to deal with as I get older.

Was it easy to cure my cancer? I have to be honest and say no. It was not easy. It took a lot of time and discipline once I figured it all out. But was it worth it? Absolutely! I feel like I never have to worry about cancer again. Now that I have gotten to the point where there is no sign of cancer in my body, it is much easier to maintain what I have accomplished than what it took to get here. I have done all the hard work. I have researched and tried all the different possibilities. If you want what I have all you have to do now is put it into action.

I would suggest that you educate yourself on a constant basis as well. Don't be afraid to try different things and see if they work. Think out of the box and be a progressive thinker. Remember the book I mentioned by Robert Barefoot and Carl J. Reich M.D. called *The Calcium Factor: The Scientific Secret of Health and Youth*? I mentioned it in an earlier chapter. I started to read this book after I had gone through everything that I have laid out in this book that you are reading. I never stop trying to learn all that I can about the physiology of the body and how to keep it healthy. Nowhere in this book do you hear me talk about calcium because I had not come across this book until just recently. The Calcium Factor is very technical but in the beginning of the book it talks about how the medical profession is resistant to changes and the way it needs to do business. The Forward and Preface talk about how nutrition is the secret to good health but the medical establishment has been very reluctant to embrace this theory just like I have mentioned in this book. Also, as I mentioned in the beginning of this book, I feel that medicine needs to go in the direction of *Preventive Medicine* rather than what I call *Reactive Medicine*. Preventive medicine is the future. In this book, the future is here for you today.

There is one last thing that I need to mention. As I have said, I have come across quite a few people that I know who have gotten cancer since I started writing this book. I told these folks about what I had discovered and that they need to try my method before they go off and try any conventional treatment. For various reasons they declined my advice. One person I knew got brain cancer and there was no way that she was going to get chemo and radiation and ruin her quality of life. I brought them all the ingredients that they needed to get started and I was even going to show them how to do it for the first few times but she sent everything back to me. She never did tell me why it was that she didn't want to get on this program. Her husband couldn't explain it either. She died 3 months later. I have another friend that elected to go with conventional chemo and radiation and she is currently in her third round of treatments. At her last checkup, doctors at a world renowned cancer treatment center found new cancer in her lymph nodes and told her that there is nothing more that they can do for her. She found a treatment center in the mid-west that accepted her as a patient. Since she gets so sick from the chemo she doesn't know if she wants to continue going down that path. She read an original manuscript of this book and for whatever reason, she won't tell us why, she does not want to try this way of a cure. I sent another person an excerpt of this book whose father had lung cancer, liver cancer and bone cancer. The doctors told him that there was nothing more they could do for him. She e-mailed me after I wrote to her to see how everything was going and she said that she, her dad and her mom (who has ovarian cancer as well) all got on this program. The dad died a month later. When I asked if they all followed this plan to the letter she told me that she and her mom did but her dad just didn't feel comfortable with some of the ingredients in this program. Wow... I could not comprehend this...

There seems to be some sort of a phenomenon going on here. I am offering people the prescription to live and they choose not to. I have been really puzzled by this. The only thing that I can think of is that people, when they learn that they have a terminal disease resolve themselves to the fact that they are going to die and once they have resolved themselves to this fact there is no turning them around. There are also those that will go through the hell of chemotherapy but will not follow this course. I know that it is because they are putting their faith and mortality in a doctor's hands but there comes a point when that doctor tells you that there is nothing more that they can do and that patient still will not embrace this program. This is probably something that will take quite some time for me to understand and figure

114

out. If you are the caregiver or family member who has purchased this book to help a loved one you may run into this same phenomenon yourself. My own family member is going through this right now. The doctors are telling them not to adopt this treatment, that it would be detrimental to the surgery and the chemotherapy. I ask you, how can natural ingredients like flaxseed oil, cottage cheese, roots and herbs in the Essiac tea and the B vitamin derivative in IP6 with Inositol be detrimental? These are all food grade natural ingredients. I don't get it…

If you are a cancer stricken patient and you have bought this book for yourself to do what I have done, I hope that you don't try to take the easy way out and you do decide to implement the steps in this book just the way I did it. And just like everything in life… If you are going to do it, do it the right way the first time and you will be so happy that you did. You can rest comfortably that chances of it coming back are going to be very slim curing yourself this way….. Cancer will not be able to survive in your body.

Cancer did not afflict you overnight. Chances are you had been living with it for quite some time before it got so bad that you finally discovered it. So, this program will not work overnight either. Don't try to take the quick and easy way out. Do what nature intended you to do to cure yourself. Don't try to shortcut this program. Follow it exactly to get the results that you are looking for. Give yourself a chance at a long healthy life and work this program… Give it six months minimum without compromise and tell me your success story.

A Journey Of A Thousand Miles Begins With A Single Step…… Lao-tzu
Time To Get Started ……

E-mail Address:
curingcancers@gmail.com

Blog Posts:
curingcancernaturally.wordpress.com

References

1. The Alkaline Acidic Handbook
     By Dr Susan E. Brown and Larry Trivieri, Jr.

2. The Calcium Factor: The Scientific Secret to Health and Youth
     By Robert R Barefoot and Carl J. Reich, M.D.

3. Ageless
     By Suzanne Somers

4. Natural Cancer Cure: The Definitive Guide To Using Dietary Supplements To Fight and Prevent Cancer

5. Testosterone for Life
     By Dr. Abraham Morgenthaler, M.D.

6. Herbal Medicine, Healing & Cancer
     By Donald R. Yance and Arlene Valentine

7. On The Origin of Cancer Cells.
     By Otto Warburg Science 1956 Feb;123:309-14.

8. The Truth About Food Grade Hydrogen Peroxide
     By: James Paul Roguski (Online Book - google this title)

9. The One Minute Cure
     By: Madison Cavanaugh

10. Wordnetweb.princeton.edu/perl/webwn

11. Prevention Magazine....

Websites

1. www.healingdaily.com/detoxification-diet/water-filtration-systems.htm)

2. www.evenbetternow.com

3. www.healthfreedom. info/Cancer%20Essiac.htm

4. www.healingdaily.com/detoxification-diet/sugar.htm

5. www.healingdaily.com/conditions/saliva-ph-test.htm

6. http://www.healingdaily.com/conditions/cancer-and-oxygen.htm

7. www.cellfood.com

8. http://acidalkalinediet.com/listofalkaline foods.pdf

9. http://www.healingdaily.com/conditions/saliva-ph-test.htm

10. www.foodgrade-hydrogenperoxide.com

11. http://www.healingdaily.com/conditions/cancer-and-oxygen.htm

12. http://www.cancure.org/ budwig_diet.htm

13. http://www.mnwelldir.org/docs/cancer1/budwig.htm

14. http://www.youtube.com/watch?v= RSoddptWL0s

15. http://jn.nutrition.org/ content/133/11/3778S.full

INDEX

A

ABM Mushroom, 62
acid reflux, 15
acidic, 49
Adrenal Glands, 13
age spots, 75
ALA
    Alpha Lipoic Acid, 63
ALAmar, 54
ALAmax CR
    antioxidant, 63
alkaline, 49, 55, 73
amino acids
    protein, 47
Anemia
    low red blood cell count, 73
Anti-Aging Doctors, 13
Apple Cider Vinegar, 55
arthritis, 49
Avemar, 54
    wheat germ derivative, 63

B

Barber, Mickey Dr., 13
Barlean's, 57
    cold pressed flax seed oil, 57
Barrett's esophagus, 15
basil cell skin cancer, 6
belladonna, 41
Bentonite, 24, 41
biopsy, 8, 20, 65
Blessed Thistle, 59
body fat, 44
Budwig
    Budwig recipe, 47, 56, 57, 59
Burdock Root,, 59

C

calcium, 49, 76
carcinogenic
    meat, 45
casein protein. *See* protein
CELLFOOD, 47, 54
CELLFOOD DNA-RNA Cell Regeneration Formula, 54, 56
cellular cleansing, 24, 55
Cellular cleansing
    essiac tea, Flor-Essence, 24
Cenegenics Medical Institute, 13
champagne, 58
Chemotherapy, 2, 70, 72, 73
chocolate
    Hershey's, 44
Chondroitin, 64
Cialis, 24
colon cleansing, 24, 38, 39, 40, 41
Co-Q-10, 64
cottage cheese, 57
CPVC plumbing, 38
Curley, Steven Dr., 8
Cyber Knife, 8
cyponate
    testosterone, 22

D

detoxify, 38, 42, 62
Dr Taub
    Dr. Harvey Taub, 8, 11
Dr. Ohhira's Professional Grade, 43

E

endocrinologist, 21
esophageal cancer, 72
Essiac tea, 24, 42, 47, 59
    Flor-Essence, 42
exercise, 51

F

Fish Oil, 64
flax seeds, 58
flaxseed oil, 57
Flor-Essence. *See* essiac tea
Flor-Essence Tea, 54, 59
Free PSA
    PSA, Free, 22

fried foods, 47
Functional Doctor, 13, 22, 68

G

GHRH
    Growth Hormone Releasing Hormone, Sermorelin, 17
Gleason Scores, 8, 66
Glucosamine, 64
glucose, 48
Great Plains Bentonite, 41

H

Hall, Douglas Dr., 13, 14, 15, 62
heavy metals, 24, 41, 42
heterocyclic amines
    HCA's, 45
HIFU Method, 7
holistic, 5
honey, 57
Human Chorionic Gonadotropin
    HCG, 18
human growth hormones
    HGH, 16
hydrogen peroxide, 54

I

immune system, 43, 49
immunity system, 75
impotence, 24
incontinence, 7, 24
Indian Rhubarb Root, 59
Inner Bark, 59
IP6 w/ Inositol, 47, 60
IP6 with Inositol, 54, 60

J

Juko Kai
    karate, 39

K

Kansius, John, 8
karate, 52
Kelp, 59
knees, 53

L

lactic acid, 49

lactic acids, 54
Laparoscopic Fundoplication, 15
Lycopene, 54, 62

M

maitake mushroom, 54
maitake Mushroom, 61
Mayo, 8, 10, 11, 15, 16, 20, 21, 22, 23, 44, 48, 50, 65, 66
MD Anderson, 8
Men's Rebuild, 38
Mintz, Alan Dr., 13

N

Natural Killer Cells, 60
Nexium, 15
Nissen Fundoplication, 15

O

Ojibwa
    Canadian Indian Tribe, 59
OncoPlex, 54, 62
organic, 45, 47
Organic, 45
oxygen, 54
oxygenating, 52

P

Pantothenic Acid, 16
Pearson, Dirk, 13
pH, 49, 50, 54, 55, 75
polycyclic aromatic hydrocarbons, 45
pomegranate extract, 54, 57
Pomegranate Extract, 58
Potassium Bicarbonate, 55
Prilosec, 15
probiotic, 43
prostate cancer, 4, 6, 7, 9, 10, 11, 13, 20, 22, 25, 40, 65, 68, 72, 75
Prostate Specific Antigen
    PSA, PSA Tests, PSA Scores, 9
prostatectomy, 7, 8, 10, 24, 61
protein, 45, 46
PSA, 9, 10, 20, 21, 22, 24, 65, 66, 67, 68
PSA test, 21, 65, 66
purified water, 47

R

Radiation, 2, 7, 72
Red Clover, 59

Red meat
    red meat, 45
relaxation, 52
Rene Caisse, 59
Resveratrol, 54, 64
Rodriguez, Dr., 20

S

saliva test, 14, 16
Saw Palmetto, 62
Selenium, 64
Sermorelin, 17, 18
    GHRH, Growth Hormone Releasing Hormone, 17
Shaw, Sandy, 13
Sheep Sorrel, 59
skin cancer, 23, 40
Slippery Elm, 59
Somers, Suzanne, 16, 19, 79
Sonne's 7, 41
steroids, 17
stress, 52
subcutaneous, 17
sugar, 44, 48, 49, 50, 54, 58, 73, 75
sulphurated protein, 57
sulphurated protein recipe
    Budwig Protocol, 11

T

Taub
    Dr. Harvey Taub, 8, 10, 11
testosterone, 16, 17, 18, 20, 21, 22, 38, 65, 66, 67, 68
    cream, injections, 16, 17
Thrombocytopenia
    low platelet count, 73

V

Viagra, 24

W

water
    tap water, well water, 17, 18, 38, 41, 42, 47, 48, 54, 55
water molecule, 55
Watercress, 59
Whey protein, 46, *See* protein

Y

Yerba Prima, 38
yoga, 52

www.ingramcontent.com/pod-product-compliance
Lightning Source LLC
Chambersburg PA
CBHW051545170526
45165CB00002B/886